STAY
Sharp!

DR GARETH MOORE

Bestselling author of *The Penguin Book of Puzzles*
and *The Ordnance Survey Puzzle Book*

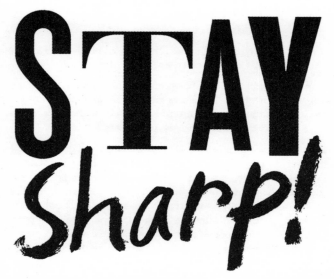

STAY *Sharp!*

Advice, Puzzles and Activities
to keep our brains active in later life

GREEN TREE

LONDON · OXFORD · NEW YORK · NEW DELHI · SYDNEY

GREEN TREE
Bloomsbury Publishing Plc
50 Bedford Square, London, WC1B 3DP, UK

BLOOMSBURY, GREEN TREE and the Green Tree logo are trademarks of
Bloomsbury Publishing Plc

First published in Great Britain 2019

A catalogue record for this book is available from the British Library

Library of Congress Cataloguing-in-Publication data has been applied for

ISBN: HB: 978-1-4729-6169-3; eBook: 978-1-4729-6171-6

2 4 6 8 10 9 7 5 3 1

Typeset in Archer by Newgen KnowledgeWorks Pvt. Ltd., Chennai, India

Printed and bound in Great Britain by CPI Group (UK) Ltd., Croydon, CR0 4YY

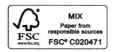

To find out more about our authors and books visit www.bloomsbury.com
and sign up for our newsletters

Contents

Introduction

Your brain changes every day, and it's a good thing it does or otherwise you wouldn't be able to learn, or do pretty much anything at all. But not all changes are good, and as we age our brains start to decline. Most of the time we don't notice this, since our greater experience of life can offset any reduction in our raw abilities. But one change we *can* observe is a reduction in our memory abilities, so let's start with that.

You might remember what you did yesterday, but what about a week ago, or a month ago? What did you do on this day five years ago? Unless you can work it out from a long-established routine, or the day was particularly memorable for some other reason, the chances are that you don't know. This isn't a change with age, however, but part of your brain's natural process of forgetting.

Why do we forget?

Forgetting things is the brain's way of allowing you to focus on what's important in life. When it comes to memory, your brain doesn't always get right what's important and what isn't – but the chances are that you do remember parts of the *most* important days of your life. Your brain will have used your unusually high emotion on those days to identify their importance, and you may well have gone over those memories many times, further reinforcing them.

But what about day-to-day life? What about remembering your hotel room number, flight time, or what it was you originally went to the supermarket to buy? Do you sometimes forget why you just got up and went to the kitchen, or what you wanted to watch on TV? Life is full of forgetfulness, and it's perfectly normal to forget these things from time to time. We all do it.

Getting older

As we get older, however, there is a general decline in both short-term memory abilities and our ability to learn and recall information over the longer term. And, just to add insult to injury, there is also a decline in our speed of thought, our ability to pay attention, and our general sensory perception.

Smarter living

If life brings these inevitable declines then what's this book all about? Well, luckily, there are many things you can do to help your brain. For example, there are various methods you can use to make it easier to remember things that you don't want to forget. We'll introduce a range of such techniques in this book, all of which have the potential to help reduce the memory-related effects of ageing. We'll also see why simply making better conscious use of your memory can make a real difference.

We'll talk about looking after your brain in order to limit the effects of age-related decline, and consider why it's important to keep on learning for as long as possible. Along the way we'll take a look at brain training, and find out what it is and whether it's something you should do. We'll cover everything from exercise and diet through to dealing with life's little (and not so little) problems. We'll also discover just how closely tied your physical and mental health are, and why it's critically important to eat a balanced diet.

What we'll achieve

As you progress through this book you'll learn a bit about the structure of your brain and your memories as you go, but these are steps on the journey to the ultimate target: a brighter, better you. Just like everyone else, you will still continue to forget things from time to time, but you'll have more control over the things you 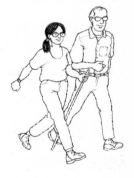 really *want* to remember, and you'll be better able to look after the whole of your brain.

What makes this book special

I've written several previous books focusing on brain training and memory, but this one is unique. First of all, it's aimed at someone who has already gone through life's more formative experiences, so we won't talk about learning for exams, for example, or dealing with peer pressure. Secondly, in this book I take a joined-up approach to the subject that allows me to cover many related aspects of your mental well-being, rather than focusing on a single aspect such as memory loss.

A further unique feature of this book is that it includes a wide range of specially designed puzzles, all of which I have written to help complement the content and to give you the chance to immediately put into practice some of the things we've just covered in the preceding pages. These are carefully tuned for the target readership of this book, based on my experience in having written many other books of brain-training puzzles, with overall sales well into the millions. These books have earned me plaudits such as 'Britain's King of Puzzles' (the *Sun*) and 'One of Britain's most trusted brain trainers' (the *Sunday Telegraph*).

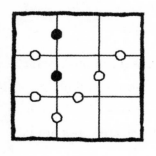

The puzzles form a core part of the book, and in order to gain the full benefit, I recommend that you don't skip over them. Even if you aren't sure you can complete them all, give each of them at least a quick try – you can always come back to them later as your confidence grows. As you'll read in later chapters, challenging yourself with the type of puzzles I've included is a great way to help look after your brain.

The puzzles can be solved in any order you like, and the rest of the book is written so it can be dipped into as you please. That said, the book also forms a progressing narrative if read through from start to finish, so your first mental challenge is to choose the reading method that works best for you!

Meet your brain

What exactly will we cover in this book? Well, we'll start by introducing you to your brain. Despite its absolutely fundamental nature to our very being, most of us are surprisingly unaware of what's going on inside our skulls. Learning just a little about how the brain works will be helpful in later chapters when we start to talk about what we can do to look after it.

After you've seen how your brain is structured, we'll talk about ageing and how your brain changes throughout your life, then take a look at some of the science in this area. We'll also discuss the impact of fitness and lifestyle on your brain.

Given that your brain can continue to change throughout your life, we'll take a look at brain training, and discuss whether it can live up to all of the claims that are often made of it. Which activities, if any, can help you in your day-to-day life, and how does their effectiveness vary with age?

We'll then be ready to move on to talk about memory in detail. What exactly is it? What are the different types of memory, and are there different types of memory loss too? We'll look at what we can do to prevent memory loss, and the importance of making greater deliberate use of your memory. We'll also cover a range of memory-related topics, such as tips for remembering a to-do list, and a method to help with memorising people's names – and then we'll try out our new skills with some memory exercises.

Build your brain

It's tempting to think of learning as something you once did at school, but in reality it's something we should all be doing every day. We'll explain just why lifelong learning is something we should all be striving for – and the mental benefits it brings, beyond simply the knowledge itself. We'll use various word and language puzzles to practise some key skills, and look at what you can do in your day-to-day life to continue to enrich your thought processes and exercise your brain more effectively.

Life is full of ups and downs, and something that many of us find difficult from time to time is staying positive – so we'll talk about this in detail, covering areas such as self-confidence and dealing with regrets. We'll see why being able to cope with these effectively is so important for your brain. We'll also use logic and reasoning puzzles to illustrate just how powerful your brain is, demonstrating that you are far more mentally flexible than you might otherwise have guessed.

Concentration and attention both become harder to maintain as we grow older, so we'll devote an entire chapter to this topic. This will include tips on gaining and maintaining focus, and avoiding distractions. We'll also talk about just how important it is to be paying proper attention if you really want to remember something. We'll include puzzles that require you to be concentrating to make progress, so you can test your focus right away. And we'll also consider some general techniques on getting started on particularly tough tasks – which should also help with the puzzles!

Care for your brain

Without your brain, you wouldn't be able to do anything, and yet how much time do you spend looking after it? It's important to care for yourself, so we'll talk about how your mood and feelings affect your brain, and the type of activities that your brain particularly enjoys. We'll also talk about sleep – and why it's so critical to both memory and your health – and how it's never too late in life to try new things. Mindfulness and meditation will be briefly covered, and we'll include a range of creative tasks to help you try out some of the techniques introduced in the chapter.

Throughout life you learn a wide range of skills, so we'll look at why it's wise to keep expanding our abilities, even as we age – including both physical and mental skills. We'll look at how a change of perspective, both literally and metaphorically, can work wonders, and how setting achievable goals can help make life more rewarding. Reasoning and number puzzles that require clever thinking to solve will help illustrate these points.

Finally, we'll have some concluding thoughts, and then end the book with solutions to the puzzles that went before. But, long before you solve that final puzzle, you will be well on the way to taking much better care of your brain – and better able to make good use of your memory. You'll be ready to go beyond the pages of this book, armed with the day-to-day determination to *Stay Sharp!*

1 The Brain and How it Works

Welcome to your brain!

Okay, so you might not be a new owner, but the chances are that your brain is a bit like the engine in your car or the electronics in your phone. You're glad they work, but you don't know the details.

When it comes to cars and electronics, you can get by without understanding what's going on. You can take them to be serviced – or even replace them, if necessary. But you don't need to be a brain surgeon to know that these aren't options for your mind – you've just got the one brain, and it's up to you to look after it! No one else can.

Time for an overhaul

When your car, phone or brain were new, they took care of themselves. They just worked. But now, as they start to age, it's time for some maintenance. Where do we start? How *do* we look after our brains? We know a bit about keeping physically fit, and have a rough idea of what a sensible diet is, but why does no one ever tell us how to look after our brain? It's so important, and yet we rarely stop to think about looking after it.

Part of the problem is that – perhaps like a car engine or a computer circuit board – most people have only the vaguest of ideas how their brain works. And we can't look after them properly, let alone fix problems, if we don't understand them.

Hello, brain

So, what's going on upstairs? Inside the mighty powerhouse that is your brain – the most impressive machine in the known universe – how exactly *do* you think thoughts, and why is it that you remember some things so easily while others are much tougher to learn? And, when something goes wrong, what can we do about it?

Well, the truth is that our brains came pre-installed, and we humans haven't yet worked out all of the operating details – but we're on the way, and what we do know so far has the potential to be incredibly useful. In fact, there are things you should know about your brain that could transform the rest of your life – they are *that* important.

So yes, we don't yet know the full details of how your brain works, and won't for many years yet to come, but that doesn't mean that what we *do* know isn't useful.

An inside look

Let's start at the beginning, with a bit of basic brain biology, and learn about how your brain is built. Even just having a rough understanding of what's going on can be helpful, and perhaps give some sense of just how complex your brain really is.

In this chapter we're going to:

> ► Start by talking about the cells that make up your brain, and how they're connected together. This knowledge is useful because it helps to understand just *why* what you eat, what drugs you take, and how fit you are can all directly affect every part of your brain.

> ► Next up, we'll take a look at how the whole of your brain is divided up into different areas, with different functions and abilities. This is important to know, because it helps explain many of the stranger behaviours of the brain, such as how ideas can suddenly appear fully formed.

> ► After this, we'll walk through some of the implications of what you've just learned, in terms of areas such as

multitasking, speed of thought, competing impulses and more.

▶ Finally, we'll look at some of the most fundamental ways you can look after your brain, now you understand a bit more about what it takes to make it work.

Cells: building blocks for brains

Cells are the basic building blocks of life. Every animal on earth evolved from early single-cell creatures, and every human on the planet grew from a single cell at conception into the amazingly complex person that you are today.

Each and every part of your body is constructed from millions of cells. Your brain is no exception, and mostly consists of two different types of cell:

▶ **Neurons** – of which there are a staggering 100 billion in your brain, or thereabouts;

▶ **Glial cells** – astonishingly, our brains contain as many as 1 *trillion* glial cells, which provide support for the neurons.

Brain wiring

Every neuron is connected on average to 1,000 other neurons, resulting in a total of around 100 trillion wiring connections in your brain. That's an incredibly hard number to visualise, so, to put it into perspective, consider this: if you were to examine one of those connections every second, it would take you over 3 *million* years just to look at them all – once!

Now, consider that almost all of these connections can be modified and adapted as you learn – and sometimes rerouted, removed or even newly constructed – and you start to gain some indication of just how powerful and flexible your brain really is.

So what exactly *is* a neuron?

A neuron is a specialist type of cell that can receive inputs from a large number of other neurons, make a decision based on those inputs, and then send the resulting decision on to a large number of further neurons. You can imagine it as a very small and specialist computer, and the way in which each individual neuron works is every bit as intricate and involved as a computer – if not more so. And, to carry the analogy even further, not only can you change the software that the neuron is running, but sometimes you can also plug it in differently so it is connected to different other computers. Neurons are reprogrammed all the time, as you learn skills and behaviours, and gain memories.

As each neuron receives and transmits signals to and from other neurons, it is the flow, speed and duration of these signals that corresponds to your behaviour, and probably your current thoughts too. Similarly, the way in which the neurons are connected together, and the varying strengths of these connections, corresponds with *who* you are. It's a funny thought, to imagine your mind as a collection of cells and electrical currents, wired together into a hugely complex machine, but that's what your brain is. However, while your brain may represent the sum of all your knowledge, it's likely to be the various electrical signals and currents in your brain that represent your consciousness.

Who am I?

Are we really entirely represented by the connections in our brains? It's certainly possible. But the brain uses so much energy that we can't be sure how all of it is used, and one theory suggests that continual loops of signals that stay entirely within the brain may account for some of it. These could be used for maintaining not just neural pathways but actual states of being, which ultimately could account for aspects of your conscious being.

Connecting neurons

Neurons connect together, and they do this via specialist parts of the cell. Each neuron consists of an input area, made up of tree-like branches called dendrites, and a long nerve fibre, the axon, which acts as an output area and ends in a series of projections – and which in turn connect to other neurons. It looks a bit like this:

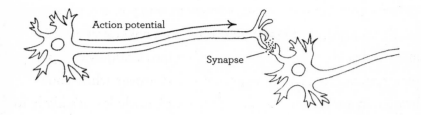

Action potential

Synapse

In the middle of the neuron is the soma, which contains the core of the cell, known as its nucleus, and is the principal 'computer' responsible for deciding whether to send a signal on to the next neuron or not. The places where neurons connect together, from the axon of one neuron to the dendrite of another, are called synapses. More specifically, it is the space between them that *is* the synapse.

Sending signals

To communicate with one another, neurons generate small electrical pulses called action potentials. These can last for as little as one millisecond, and carry only around a tenth of a volt. They travel out from the neuron along the axon, and each time they reach a synaptic connection they trigger a signal on the adjoining dendrite of another neuron. It's a bit like zapping your neighbouring friends with a tiny electrical prod. And then, like each friend, the next neuron might react – or it might decide to ignore the prod. In fact, the prod might make your friend *less* likely to do something. It depends on your friend; and in your brain, it depends on the neuron. These signals can both stimulate and inhibit other responses in the brain.

Keeping it working

As we've already seen, there are also glial cells in your brain, and they far outnumber the neurons. Given their quantity, you might think that the glial cells are even more critical to our thinking processes than the neurons, but – according to our current understanding of the brain – their main function is to support the neurons. They do this primarily by supplying and regulating the flow of chemicals to the neurons, and also by building insulation around your brain's wiring to help make it faster and more durable. This leaves the neurons to do all of the heavy mental lifting.

Bearing in mind that there are around 1 trillion glial cells, and that one of their key functions is to supply necessary chemicals to the neurons, this gives you some idea of just how important it is to make sure that you eat a healthy diet and stay fit. Having this quantity of cells shows how critical their role is, and yet their ability to supply those nutrients is dependent on your heart's physical ability to pump blood around your body efficiently. Without good fitness and a good diet, the glial cells won't have the supplies they need to keep your neurons working properly. And, if that happens, you either fail to think as well as you could, or your neurons simply die – and most of them can't ever regrow.

So we need to be physically fit, and eat a balanced diet, in order to ensure a regular supply of the necessary chemicals – including oxygen for power – for the many cells that make up our brain. As we'll see later in the book, there's also considerable evidence that maintaining your fitness helps maintain brain function into later life.

Synaptic connections

Sometimes the synaptic connection between two neurons is tiny, even by microscopic standards, and electrical signals can jump across it directly. Most of the time, however, there is a small gap, and the brain needs to do something clever to connect them. And the way it does this is by using chemicals that are collectively known as neurotransmitters.

Neurotransmitters diffuse across the gap from one neuron to the next, where eventually they reach a receptor on an adjoining dendrite. This incoming chemical signal can then either encourage or discourage the receiving neuron from generating an action potential of its own. This neuron will in turn decide whether to generate its own action potential based on the information gathered from all of its inputs.

Complex connections

The level of complexity in this system is staggering. Not only are there exceptions to the types of connection described above, but there are many different types of neurotransmitter, each with its own behaviour and its own receptors. For some neurotransmitters, the effect on the neuron might not just be momentary but could be longer-lasting. And different neurotransmitters penetrate the brain in different ways, too: some will also affect neighbouring neurons, while others flood large areas of the brain, significantly changing our behaviour.

A message in a bottle

You can imagine neurotransmitters as little messages in a bottle, which are thrown into a sea. The sending neuron triggers the release of them into the synapse, and then they float across that synapse until eventually they reach the other side. When they reach the receiving neuron, they trigger an electric signal on its dendrite.

This analogy works quite well, because it helps highlight some of the potential problems:

► What if you don't have enough bottles to throw?

► What if there are already too many bottles in the sea?

► What if you have the wrong types of bottle?

And indeed, these are all problems your brain can have, once you substitute 'neurotransmitter' for 'bottle'.

The analogy also helps because you can imagine how much slower these signals are than those sent via direct electrical connections, and how much the behaviour of your brain depends on a regular supply of the desired neurotransmitters.

Your nervous system

Neurons are found not just in your brain, but also throughout the entirety of your nervous system. This covers not just the central nervous system, which is the part of your nervous system that is encased in bone – including both your brain and your spinal cord – but also the peripheral nervous system that reaches to the extremes of your body. In a sense, you have a few bits of your brain stretched out across your body, so that you can control what it does and keep up to date on its current situation.

Specialised neurons connect from your spinal cord to key parts of your body – where, for example, they send signals to certain muscles to expand or contract, or receive pain signals when you hurt yourself. The longest such connection is an axon that travels from a neuron in the base of your spine all the way to your toes – which can therefore be over 1 metre (3 feet) long. That's a big cell! Mind you, that's nothing compared to a giraffe, which has some neurons that contain axons running several metres along the entire length of its neck.

Drugs for the brain

Some drugs work by changing the balance of neurotransmitters in the brain – antidepressants, for example, increase the quantity of certain neurotransmitters within synapses. This is intended to redress what are thought to be imbalances that are connected with depression. This in turn changes the decisions made by the connected neurons, since they receive inputs that would otherwise have been suppressed by a lack of neurotransmitters in the neighbouring synapse.

Just send me a message

Not all of your body is connected directly to the nervous system, however – other parts are controlled chemically via the bloodstream, with these chemical messages being received by the glands. A special part of the brain, known as the pituitary gland, sticks out past the blood-brain barrier, releasing these chemicals – hormones – that tell other parts of your body how to behave. For example, it releases an anti-diuretic hormone that helps control blood pressure, by changing the behaviour of both the kidney and blood vessels. It also controls the amount of water you urinate, ensuring you keep enough for your body to function.

These chemical messages are much slower to move around your body, which is why it can take a long time for some signals to be received. They are also received by the brain from your body – for example, part of the mechanism of letting your brain know you're full after eating involves a hormone produced by the digestive system. This takes a while to make its way to your brain in sufficient quantities, which is one reason why it's good to eat slowly – and wait 20 minutes before deciding on whether you really do want dessert.

Learning

Your brain is full of neurons that connect together, and the way these neurons are programmed represents all of your skills and memories. But what if you want to learn something new?

Strengthening connections

When your brain learns, it does so by strengthening the connections between certain neurons, and possibly weakening that between others. Although on a neuron-by-neuron level there may be no immediately obvious pattern, the overall effect of this is to link concepts together that fit together, and to separate those things that the brain now knows don't go together. We'll see in later chapters how memories are strengthened by associating them with one another.

The brain modifies these connections in various ways, such as by altering the balance of neurotransmitters in a synapse, or by creating additional receptors on a neuron so it is more sensitive. Different methods have different degrees of durability, which goes some way to explaining why many memories fade so quickly – chemical changes in the balance of neurotransmitters will sometimes slowly revert back to their original state if not reinforced by more permanent changes in the brain.

Making new connections

Your brain also learns by rewiring itself, adding connections between neurons. This means that, as you grow older, you are likely to have a greater proportion of synapses relative to neurons than you did when you were younger.

This rewiring generally only happens on a local scale, however. Although there are many long-distance connections in your brain, these are thought to be entirely formed while you are young and your brain is still developing. This is probably why certain behaviours, such as the ability to easily distinguish certain speech sounds, are most easily developed in the first years of life. Developing these skills later is not always impossible, but is considerably harder than it would be as a young infant.

Pruning connections

Your brain doesn't just *add* connections – it also removes the ones you don't use. So, if you were to sit around all day watching particularly mindless TV shows, and not challenge yourself in any real way, you really would lose certain abilities you might otherwise have retained. This also accounts for the loss of previously long-lasting memories, once you cease to find them useful.

Why does your brain remove connections, if they aren't causing any problems? Well, your brain continually learns from your behaviour, so if you are stuck in a dull routine, it will start to optimise itself to fit with that dull routine – it doesn't judge you, but just does what it observes best suits your behaviour. Luckily, even in this situation your brain is still smart enough to learn anew – so even later in life you can teach it new tricks that can help counteract the effect of neglect in earlier years; but you will find it tougher than you would have done some years before.

Energy consumption

You might wonder why your brain would bother to discard sections that you are not using. While one reason is no doubt to make better use of space, an important further reason is that your brain uses an *enormous* amount of the body's energy – in fact, it uses about 20 per cent of all your energy, despite accounting for only around 5 per cent of your total mass. So, on an evolutionary scale, where until very recently humans could never be sure of having enough food, it was important for your brain to use no more energy than it needed.

It is predicted that it will take a long time – perhaps 100,000 years – for human evolution to have a chance to adapt us to a life where food is in plentiful supply; and it could be substantially longer, since modern medicine may well slow down natural selection.

The shape of your brain

Do you know what your brain looks like? You probably have a vague idea, based on pictures you might have seen, that it is grey and soft, and is wrinkled like a giant walnut. That's an accurate description, but that's just the top surface of the brain – the cerebral cortex. This is the most evolved part of your brain, where all your cleverest thinking is done. But it doesn't all look like that.

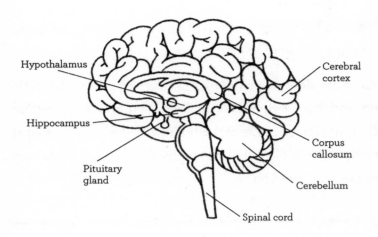

Hypothalamus

Cerebral cortex

Hippocampus

Corpus callosum

Pituitary gland

Cerebellum

Spinal cord

The outermost brain

The most complex neuronal networks are found in the outermost part of your brain, most of which is taken up by the cerebrum (which includes the cerebral cortex). In fact, the cerebrum contains around 90 per cent of your brain's neurons.

A brain of two halves

The cerebrum is divided into two hemispheres, one on each side of your body, which are primarily connected via the axons of what is known as the corpus callosum. You don't need to remember the name of the connecting part, but it's useful to know that your brain has two hemispheres. Generally speaking, the left side of your brain deals with the right side of your body, and the right side of your brain deals with the left side of your body – but it is a bit more complex when it comes to your eyes, where your brain splits its visual processing based on the left- and right-hand *sides* of each eye.

There is considerable similarity between the two sides of the brain, and many behaviours occur on both sides. For certain skills, however, one side of the brain will specialise in that skill, but whether it is the left or right side can in some cases vary from person to person.

Left- and right-brained people

It is often claimed that people are either left- or right-brained, meaning that they have a bias to using one particular side of their brain. This is based on research from the early twentieth century, which found that damage to one side of the head could cause specific skills to be lost. Since certain skills are localised on particular sides, the idea arose that if you favoured one side then you would be better at the skills located on that side of the brain.

Even allowing for the fact that some skills can be found on different sides of the brain in different people, the truth is that both sides of your brain work together all the time, so the idea that you are biased towards one side is not true. This is great news for anyone who was ever told that the way their brain was wired meant that they 'weren't creative', or that they could never get better at maths! You have the capacity to learn these skills – just like everyone else.

Each hemisphere is divided into four areas:

► The frontal lobe, which carries out the higher mental processes such as planning for the future, and deciding what to wear today. It's located at the front part of the brain, and it's what makes you *you*.

► The temporal lobe, which is just behind your temples, and among other tasks is responsible for dealing with information received by your ears.

► The occipital lobe, at the lower back of the cerebrum, which is the area responsible for dealing with information that is received by the eyes.

► The parietal lobe, at the upper back of the cerebrum, and which deals with combining information from all of your senses, including handling your ability to pay attention to something.

The cerebral cortex

The outermost part of the cerebrum is the topmost part of your brain, the cerebral cortex, which wraps around all but the bottom of your brain. It has a wrinkled texture that allows it to pack in more neurons than could be fitted if it were stretched out flat. In fact, if it *were* stretched out flat, it would cover about 1½ square metres (16 square feet).

The cerebral cortex handles your most advanced behaviours, including your ability to be conscious of your own existence and therefore fully aware of yourself as a person. It provides your capacity for intelligent thought, complex language skills, creativity and learning. It also handles voluntary physical actions – although involuntary ones, such as an automatic pulling back of your hand when it unexpectedly feels pain, are triggered elsewhere.

White matter

Beneath the grey matter of the cerebral cortex lies the bulk of the cerebrum, made up primarily of white matter – this is packed with long-distance connections between neurons. It really does look white, and this colour comes from the myelin, formed by all those glial cells, which is used to coat and protect important, long-lasting connections within the brain.

Other parts of the cerebrum

At the bottom of the cerebrum lies a set of brain structures referred to as the limbic system. These combine higher mental functions with more primitive ones – and, to give one example, are responsible for providing you with pleasure when you eat certain foods. Some parts of the limbic system include:

▶ The hippocampus, which plays a key role in consolidating memory, among other functions. See also chapter 2.

▶ The basal ganglia, which handles a range of behaviours, including the learning of procedural memories such as how to ride a bicycle.

▶ The olfactory bulb, which deals with your sense of smell.

▶ The amygdala, which deals with emotions. Its physical proximity to the hippocampus perhaps provides a clue as to why emotions are so important in storing memories.

▶ The thalamus, which acts as a connection between the cerebrum and other parts of the brain, helping coordinate information between different areas of the brain.

▶ The hypothalamus, which deals with various bodily functions such as body temperature, thirst and hunger.

The cerebellum

At the lower back of the brain sits an evolutionarily older part known as the cerebellum. It coordinates the behaviour of your muscles, following instructions from the cerebral cortex about how you want to move your body. For example, the cerebellum allows you to move your hand smoothly without having to consciously think about each individual movement along the way.

In order to work, the cerebellum also receives information from the cerebral cortex about what your various senses are perceiving, so it can know what is required of it. It is therefore involved in balance and maintaining a particular posture, too.

The brainstem

The most primitive part of the brain is right at the bottom, in the centre, forming the lower parts of the brainstem, which connects from the base of the brain into the top of the spinal cord. It handles the most basic animal behaviours, such as breathing. This is also why you can't just forget to breathe – you don't need to remember, since it's a built-in behaviour.

Multitasking

Unconscious thought accounts for far more than our relatively unevolved responses, and extends right through to our higher consciousness. In fact, no matter how much we may believe we can multitask, studies have shown that we are capable only of consciously thinking of one thing at a time. We may create the illusion of thinking of multiple things, but in fact we simply become good at switching from one task to another with relatively little confusion (although often we are not quite as good at this as we think we are!). But this does not mean that we cannot *unconsciously* be thinking about something else.

Given the enormous complexity of our brains, and the duplication between the left and right hemispheres, it is entirely possible for complex thoughts to be being considered without us being consciously aware of them. Just take a moment to think about all the times that the solution to a problem suddenly came to you, quite possibly even when you weren't immediately just thinking about it. How could that happen, unless your unconscious brain had continued to think about it even after your conscious mind had moved on?

Considerable unconscious thought also takes place while you sleep. Sleep, however, is such an important subject that we will return to it in a later chapter.

Brain chemistry

Your brain relies on a wide range of chemicals to function. Many of these are used up over time, and it is important to include these chemicals in your diet, so that your brain can either use them directly or use them to synthesise other compounds it requires.

The key chemicals and elements that you need – and which must be present in the diet – can be broken down into four groups:

▶   Vitamins: organic compounds that the body requires, but which it cannot synthesise itself.

▶   Minerals: natural elements found on earth, which the body needs in order to work.

▶   Essential fatty acids: omega-3 and omega-6 polyunsaturated fatty acids.

► Essential amino acids: certain amino acids that cannot be made by the body, and which are found in various proteins.

A healthy diet

You might wonder what foods you should eat to look after your brain, especially if you've read about 'miracle' foods that make you smarter. Sadly, there is no magical panacea, and the truth is that the most important thing you can do is to make sure you have a properly balanced diet.

So long as your diet is sufficiently varied, a normal fit and healthy adult ordinarily won't require any additional dietary supplements, or special foods – and for the healthy there is little evidence that having an excess of any substance (i.e. more than the Recommended Dietary Allowance – RDA) can lead to benefits over and above the brain's standard requirements.

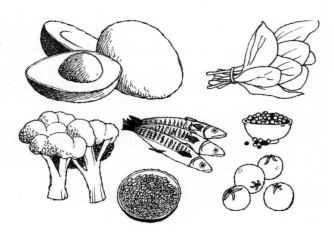

Dietary supplements

In general, there is no point in taking a supplement – such as a pill or capsule – which means that you will be ingesting considerably more than the Recommended Dietary Allowance (RDA) of a substance. The excess will either be excreted harmlessly, or will build up and potentially cause health problems – and, in either case, it has not helped you.

Vitamin supplements that contain more than the Recommended Dietary Allowance should generally be taken only if prescribed by a doctor for a specific ailment – or if they are generally advised by the medical community for a specific situation, such as pregnancy. Multivitamins, on the other hand, are a good insurance policy – specifically those which cover most of what you require each day, but which don't exceed the RDA of any particular substance. These broad-spectrum multivitamin tablets are unlikely to cause you harm, and could even considerably help you by allowing you to cope with gaps in your diet which you don't realise you have.

If you do take supplements, it's important to note that recent research has shown that most are best taken as part of a meal. When swallowed on their own, sometimes very little – if any – of the content makes it into the bloodstream.

Recently, there has been a trend for injecting vitamins and other supplements directly into the bloodstream via an intravenous (IV) drip, but this could be dangerous unless administered by a qualified medical professional, and only as approved by a doctor.

Brain food

There are some foods that are often referred to as 'brain foods', but there is little solid evidence that any specific food is better than others for healthy people. Even foods containing omega-3, as found particularly in oily fish, are certainly required by your brain but taking them in amounts beyond the RDA has not been proven to further help with cognitive function – although there is some evidence that an additional intake may help those with mild cognitive impairment.

There is, however, good evidence that extra omega-3 does provide other health benefits, and little evidence that taking extra omega-3 can cause problems, at least without taking especially excessive amounts, so adding additional oily fish or linseed to your diet is still a sensible choice. You might also think that an omega-3 supplement capsule would be a good alternative, but unfortunately these seem to be less effective – and, in fact, for some purposes there is evidence that they are not effective *at all*. So your best bet is to include omega-3 as part of a regular diet, not as a pill, if you can.

Another supplement that is sometimes recommended for a 'healthy brain' is to take extra vitamin E. Unfortunately, while some initial studies suggested that this might help prevent cognitive decline, later studies have failed to repeat these results. Also, while it is safe to take more vitamin E than you require through food, it is in general *not* considered safe to take sustained excessive vitamin E via dietary supplements. So you should do this only if recommended by a doctor.

Summary

If you've read the entirety of this chapter, congratulations! You are now the fully qualified owner of a brain, and know far more about what's going on upstairs than the majority of other people. You're ready to put it through its paces as you work your way through the rest of this book.

In particular, we've covered the structure of your brain, in terms of both its primitive regions and its more evolved outer regions, and seen how its outer layer is made up of the hugely complex cerebral cortex – which gives it its grey, wrinkled appearance. We've also seen how it is divided into hemispheres, and how different types of activity are localised in different parts of the brain.

We've also looked at how your brain works in close detail, examining the structure of the cells that make up most of your brain. We saw how they function and connect together, and saw how important it is that we do what we can to remain fit, and eat a balanced diet. We also considered how your brain learns, and saw why some memories might fade with time.

In brief

- ► Your brain has 100 billion neurons, plus around 100 trillion synaptic connections between neurons.

- ► Neurons transmit signals to one another, representing your thoughts. This behaviour can be influenced by emotions, or by drugs.

- ► Your brain learns by making and strengthening connections between neurons.

- ► If you don't make use of parts of your brain, they may be discarded.

- ► Most of your neurons are in the higher-level parts of your brain, which represent your conscious mind.

- ► The complexity of your brain, and its different evolutionary components, mean that you often have competing urges and feelings.

- ► Sometimes you have to make a conscious effort to overrule certain primitive behaviours.

▶ Your brain is capable of thinking without you being consciously aware of it.

▶ A balanced diet is critical to maintaining a healthy brain.

Coming up

In the next chapter, we'll take a look at how your brain evolves and changes over your life, with a particular focus on your memory.

2 The Changing Brain

You might think of your brain as something that doesn't really physically change throughout your adult life. Of course you continue to learn and gain new memories, but, since we can't see it, we don't know much about what happens during adulthood – so let's take a look at the story of your brain. We'll then use this knowledge to help make sense of the changes that age brings.

From baby to adult

During your first few years of life, your brain developed at a fearsome rate, building connections and learning new skills. Your brain peaked in the complexity of its neuronal wiring just before puberty and then, as you entered puberty, your brain started a process of optimisation in which it discarded as many as half of all the synaptic connections it previously had. When you consider that you have around 100 trillion connections even now, this gives some indication of the incredible changes that your brain went through as you entered teenage life.

This cleaning and tidying of your brain helped prepare you to face the adult world, and led to the strengthening and speeding-up of the remaining connections. It took a while to be complete, however, which is one reason why children are not allowed to vote, or be held to the same standards as adults.

The process of brain tidying and construction continued into your 20s, facilitating learning. And then, at about 25 years of age, you reached your mental peak – and quite possibly your physical one too. After this, your brain gently began to decline in a process that has continued ever since. What's more, this decline slowly accelerates as you age.

Don't abandon hope!

The good news is that, if you have coped with using your brain since your late 20s, there's no reason to think you aren't going to continue coping. There's no sudden change that takes place when you reach a certain age. Instead, as life continues, some of your neurons (the cells that make up your brain) will continue to die – and not be replaced – just as has been happening for all of your adult life, without much noticeable effect.

The second bit of good news is that, as we saw in the previous chapter, you have rather a lot of neurons to begin with, and the greater experience you bring to life will often compensate for any sprightliness of thought lost since you were younger. So even if a younger person can actually think *faster* than you, it is often the case that they need to think *more* to reach the same conclusion as an older person. In other words, the loss of neurons is compensated for by smarter use of those that remain.

You might think that this still sounds rather depressing, but the truth is that the natural loss of your brain cells need not cause you any substantial problems – unless, of course, it becomes accelerated by disease. You might not be as mentally agile as a much younger person, but you might well be considerably smarter.

Senior moments

Do you find yourself going into a room, then forgetting why you went into it in the first place? If you do, you're not alone. We all have these 'senior moments', and – despite the name – they have happened throughout our lives.

While it may be tempting to ascribe these to the travails of age, the truth is that they are simply due to us not paying attention to what we are doing. If it's not a very interesting task, your brain doesn't take much note of it, and you can easily forget what it was. As you age, the mundane tasks of life become more and more routine, and even *less* interesting than they once were – so you forget them more.

It's also true, however, that an older brain is more easily distracted, so it might take more conscious effort to stay focused on the present moment. But don't worry about this – as life continues, so you end up with far more memories and thoughts and ideas that could all potentially distract you!

To help avoid senior moments, you could try saying out loud (even just to yourself) what you intend to do before you do it. This will help you focus on the task, and perhaps ensure you have paid sufficient attention.

Your flexible brain

The human brain is truly remarkable for its seemingly unlimited capacity to learn. What's more, it also has the ability to make significant changes in its structure – which is often referred to as brain 'plasticity'.

Brain plasticity means that your brain has considerable capacity to adapt to new situations. For example, if you lose one of your main senses, the parts of your brain normally dealing with that sense may adapt to compensate via aspects of another sense:

► In a deaf person, for example, those areas ordinarily involved with hearing will typically assist with sign language instead.

► Or, to those who aren't blind, it seems almost impossible that patterns of raised dots could be read by the fingertips – and yet the brain of a blind person can learn to read rows of Braille characters with remarkable speed and precision.

Morse code masters

Brain plasticity isn't just useful following the loss of a sense. During the two world wars in the twentieth century, for example, signal operators learned to listen to streams of Morse code blips and bleeps until they could transcribe them as easily as if they were listening to the spoken word.

What's more, they could understand the Morse code even over terrible quality signals, full of white noise and other interference.

The brains of these Morse code masters adapted to process this additional form of language, with the fluency normally reserved for our spoken and written languages.

Hard-wired processes

Despite the brain's amazing ability to adapt, there are some parts of our brain we *can't* retrain, and these are mostly accounted for by the older parts of our brain structure, as we saw in the previous chapter. We can't learn not to breathe, for example, or teach ourselves not to feel hungry. Also, we can't completely ignore pain, just by thinking it away.

Despite the fact that some things are out of our control, however, we should not be fatalistic. We may not be able to change these physiological processes, but we may well be able to influence the parts of our brains which make higher-level decisions based on these matters.

Growing a new brain

Okay, so you can't grow a whole new brain, but we do know that small parts of it can be grown – even after you reach maturity. While it's true that most neurons which die as we age will not be replaced, there are at least *some* parts of our brain which actually *can* grow new neurons. These areas, however, are mostly associated with the storage of memories, not speed of thought.

One area of the brain where neurogenesis – the creation of new neurons – is particularly prevalent is in the hippocampus (see page 27). This part of the brain is involved with the consolidation of long-term memories, and will sometimes create new neurons if it needs to store large amounts of knowledge.

The Knowledge

Since 1865, London's black cab taxi drivers have been required to learn the layout of all of the city's many streets within over a six-mile radius of Charing Cross. On top of this, they must also learn more than 300 specific routes, *and* the points of interest that cover that entire area too – a trickier task nowadays than it once was over 150 years ago, too! They are required to learn this information in order to pass The Knowledge, a test which is a condition of being granted a licence.

Scientists, marvelling at this incredible amount of encyclopaedic knowledge that needs to be learned by a single individual, wondered if there was anything special about the brains of cabbies. What they discovered was revealing. The drivers' brains appeared perfectly normal prior to starting to learn, but by the time they were able to pass the test they had gained a considerable number of new neurons in the hippocampus.

Running out of storage space

Can you 'fill up' your brain with all of that knowledge and the skills you acquire as you age? Will you one day run out of space? Well, luckily, all the evidence suggests that the answer is a resounding no. There is no recorded case of anyone suddenly being unable to learn or remember anything new, beyond rare cases associated not with limited capacity but with specific brain injuries.

It might be the case, however, that our brains start to become cluttered with knowledge. When a computer begins to fill up its storage device, new data starts to become split all over the place in the bits of space that are still free. This is called 'fragmentation', and it makes it much slower both to store and to read from that memory. Rather than keeping everything together, the machine must now wait until it has accessed several separate areas and combined the results.

A similar fragmentation effect may start to take place in the human brain as we age too. This may particularly affect us when we try to learn things that require considerable effort across many different parts of our brain. Perhaps this is why learning foreign languages requires more concentration and persistence in later life than when we are very young, for example. There are so many complementary skills to learn, including pronunciations, spellings, grammar, meanings, listening, accents, cultural differences and so on. Perhaps fitting all of this knowledge in becomes much trickier once our brain is no longer actively developing. After all, we can't just 'delete' other bits of our brain to make way for it, so there has to be a compromise somewhere along the way.

Brain changes in later life

With the regular loss of brain cells throughout adult life, it becomes more important than ever to look after your brain as you age.

Mental exercise

In order to work around the cumulative effect of cell loss over many years, it's important to continue to challenge yourself. This means that new circuits can be created to replace those that have been damaged. And, as we saw in the previous chapter, your brain may remove parts that are no longer used, so it's important to continue to push yourself mentally, simply to retain the skills you already have.

Physical exercise

There's strong evidence that maintaining some level of exercise is important for your brain, at whatever level you are capable.

This will help ensure your body is able to deliver a steady supply of the chemicals (see pages 30–1) that your brain needs to function and maintain itself.

As you age, your body also becomes worse at regulating the flow of glucose, leading to spikes in your blood sugar that could affect your brain – and which regular exercise can help minimise. Eating foods with a lower glycaemic index can also help, since they release their sugar more slowly rather than all at once.

Day-to-day memories

Your brain becomes less good at learning in old age. It's true that you already know much of what you need to know to get through life, so this is not as critical as it might once have been, but in particular the formation of new day-to-day memories can become tougher. This especially affects those parts of life where you are going about your daily routine and not deliberately attempting to remember something.

A reduction in day-to-day memories can make life seem more confusing, particularly if you suddenly realise that you know something but can't remember where or how you learned it. Adding to this, your sense of time and place associated with the memories you do form becomes less strong. This means that it can sometimes be trickier to know if something happened recently, or whether it was longer ago.

This sense of confusion over time can make it harder to remember future appointments, and might even lead to you feeling like you are losing the plot! But in reality it's just a natural part of ageing, and you can help work around it by making an effort to consciously pay attention to events – or perhaps by keeping a diary of each day, so you reinforce and strengthen your daily memories.

Short-term memory

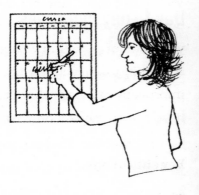

One specific change to memory in later life is that your ability to hold information in your head for short periods of time can worsen, so you might find yourself needing to write things down more often than you once did. Rather than hear a full phone number and then dial it straight away, you might need to have it read to you more slowly, dialling as you go.

As an effect of the reduced ability to remember things over the short term, older people are more likely to forget to return to a previous task after having being disturbed. This marks a return in one sense to a childlike ease of distraction, in which a previous aim is completely forgotten after switching to some other task. If this happens to you, think of it as liberating your inner child, rather than limiting your outer adult!

Memorisation techniques

It isn't all doom and gloom, however, since using certain deliberate methods to memorise information – and paying better attention – can counteract the effect of ageing. You can also, of course, simply write things down more often than you did when you were younger. Don't be afraid of people judging you for this – they'll simply think you're much more organised than they are!

We'll cover some suitable memorisation methods later in this book, but even just trying to make better conscious use of your memory – telling yourself that you want to remember something, then actively trying to do so – can lead to significant improvements. And what's more, these improvements can then have a lasting effect on your memory abilities.

Benefits of age

The brains of older people still have some advantages over those of younger adults. The wisdom you gain as you grow older doesn't just allow you to be smarter and more learned, but even extends to allowing you better control of your brain. This means you can overrule more primitive responses, and make more reasoned, sensible responses that lead to greater enjoyment of life. You can finally eschew some of the worries you might once have had.

Your age and experience allow you a more balanced view on life, meaning that over time you learn to better control your emotions. Brain scans of over-60s show how older brains have learned to respond differently to certain emotional stimuli, so your brain quite literally makes it easier to enjoy life than it once did when you were younger.

Brain illnesses

Most changes in the performance of your memory are simply the natural effects of ageing. There are some changes, however, which would cause concern, and could be early indicators of dementia – a general term for damage to the brain which causes loss of mental faculties.

Dementia is rare before the age of 65, so is typically associated with old age. It is less obvious in its early stages, so can be hard to spot, especially since changes in memory are associated with ageing in any case, as we have seen (so don't panic if you have occasional memory lapses!).

For earlier diagnosis, changes in general mood or behaviour are one indicator, and difficulty concentrating sufficiently to perform basic functions of life, such as getting dressed or cooking dinner, is another. We're not talking about forgetting you made a cup of tea – this is more serious stuff. The good news, such as it is, is that it often progresses slowly over a number of years, with average survival times of several to a dozen years – although some people will survive much longer than that.

Dementia

The most common forms of dementia are:

► Alzheimer's disease, which is the single most frequent cause of dementia, with more than 850,000 sufferers in the UK alone. The initial symptoms will depend on the part of the brain first affected, but significant changes in mental ability or personality are examples of changes that would be of potential concern. Interestingly, smarter people sometimes appear to have a slower onset of Alzheimer's, but unfortunately, this is then followed by a more sudden, apparently faster loss of abilities. This is because these people had built multiple ways of thinking the same thought, so when they first lost parts of their brains they were better able to compensate and slow the impact (but not the progress) of the disease – until the damage finally became so significant that they were no longer able to work around the loss of cognitive function, meaning that it appeared as a sudden, seemingly faster, decline.

Because it is relatively common, a lot of research is being done into the possible causes of Alzheimer's disease in the hope that it could one day be prevented, or halted once diagnosed. The disease itself progresses via two mechanisms: firstly, the accumulation of a certain protein in the synapses which would normally be broken down, but which in an Alzheimer's patient will instead accumulate and kill the neuronal connections; and, secondly, a breakdown in the behaviour of the neurons themselves, where they cease to function correctly.

► Vascular dementia, which affects around 150,000 people in the UK. As the name implies, this disease stems from a problem with blood flow to the brain, which causes either small or large parts of the brain to die. This can be caused as the result of a stroke, or a series of smaller strokes, although a disease that affects the blood vessels within the brain can also have the same effect. It is also common for it to occur at the same time as Alzheimer's. The progress of vascular dementia can sometimes be slowed down, or even halted, if it is diagnosed early enough. High blood pressure is often a contributing factor.

► Lewy Body Dementia, which affects more than 100,000 people in the UK, and involves unwanted structures forming inside neurons, which then leads to the death of those cells. Symptoms are varied, as with all forms of dementia, but may include hallucinations and periods of alertness that mix unexpectedly with periods of sleepiness or periods of confusion.

▶ Frontotemporal dementia (also known as Pick's disease), which is more common in those aged from 45 to 65, with possible symptoms including personality changes and inappropriate social behaviour, such as being tactless or making inappropriate jokes, as well as other issues such as being unusually obsessive. The disease results in unwanted proteins forming in neurons in the frontal and temporal lobes, causing the neurons to die. Around 20,000 people in the UK currently have this form of dementia.

Brush your teeth!

Recent studies have suggested that gum disease could be a significant cause of dementia, with the spread of bacteria from the mouth into the brain. So, make sure you brush your teeth twice a day, and

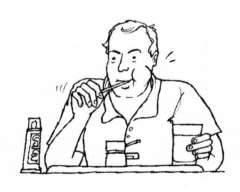

go to the dentist if you have oral issues that are waiting to be addressed. You should also go to the dentist regularly, anyway.

Other brain diseases

► Parkinson's disease is another disease that affects the brain over a series of years, leading to shaking limbs, slow movement and difficulty in moving muscles, as well as various other potential problems. Around 125,000 people in the UK have this disease, which is thought to be caused by a combination of genetic and environmental factors. It is most common in those over 50, and men are slightly more at risk than women. Parkinson's disease cannot be cured, but in many cases it can be controlled so that sufferers can still enjoy a reasonable quality of life and a fairly normal life expectancy.

► Diabetes is a disease that does not directly impact the brain, but can lead to highs or lows in the body's blood sugar level. This in turn can cause damage to the small blood vessels in the brain, leading to vascular dementia, as described in the previous section.

► Another type of brain illness is mild cognitive impairment. This is a term that refers to changes in the brain's ability which do not significantly interfere with everyday life, but which are unexpected and beyond those which are naturally associated with ageing. Examples include becoming confused when undertaking tasks that would previously not have caused any trouble, such as calculating a tip for a waiter, or forgetting recent information which would previously have been recalled with ease, such as a conversation from earlier that day. Mild cognitive impairment does not always lead to dementia – in about 50 per cent of cases the symptoms get no worse, or even go away. But because it can be triggered by various medicines, or even by stress, it can be difficult to diagnose correctly.

Preventing brain illnesses

Nothing is certain in life, but there are steps you can take to decrease your chances of being affected by dementia or other diseases of the brain. These include:

▶ Ensuring you eat a healthy and balanced diet;

▶ Staying physically fit, with regular exercise such as a brisk walk, swimming or cycling;

▶ Doing your best to keep a healthy blood pressure;

▶ Maintaining a healthy weight;

▶ Avoiding excessive alcohol consumption;

▶ Not smoking;

- ► Seeking early treatment for any health issues, including depression;

- ► Ensuring regular, good-quality social interaction;

- ► Continually challenging yourself mentally, such as by reading widely – or doing puzzles such as those found in this book.

Summary

In this chapter we covered a great many changes that can affect your brain throughout your life. After its initial rapid growth, your brain peaks at about age 25 and then there is a graceful decline throughout the rest of your life – which unfortunately does accelerate with age. Fortunately, however, there are a number of things you can do to counteract the effects of ageing, and you also gain wisdom, which can balance the loss in raw thinking speed.

We looked at how amazingly flexible your brain is, and how it can adapt to new circumstances. We looked at the storage of memories, and saw that you won't run out of space but that some types of memory do become harder to form as you age. We also saw how physical exercise and other activities can help keep your brain in much better condition, and some of the brain illnesses that can affect people – as well as ways to help improve your chances of avoiding these.

In brief

- ► Your brain develops until your mid-20s, and then starts to decline.

- ► Age and experience can compensate for a loss of brain cells caused by age.

- ► Your brain has a remarkable capacity to learn, and even create new neurons in some areas of the brain.

- ► Your brain can't 'fill up', no matter how much you know.

- ► You must continually challenge your brain as you age.

- ► It's essential to stay as fit as you can, to look after your brain.

- ► It's tougher learning in later life, which can lead to confusion.

- ► Many people find life a bit less stressful, and more enjoyable, as they age.

- ► Various illnesses can impact on your mental abilities.

► There are certain things you can do to improve your odds of not being impacted by these diseases.

Coming up

In the next chapter, we'll look in much more detail at some of the things you can do to help keep your brain fit.

3 Keeping Your Brain Fit

You have only one brain, and the responsibility is all yours to look after it.

That's all very well and good, but *how* exactly do you do that? Should you do a crossword every day, or take up sudoku; or should you stop watching TV and go and write a book?

Well, the truth is that there is no magic panacea that will keep your brain in tip-top shape, but rather a whole host of things you can do to look after it:

- ► Challenge yourself;

- ► Eat healthily;

- ► Be as fit as you can.

The second two of these are somewhat beyond the scope of this book, beyond the general dietary advice given earlier, so in this chapter we're going to focus on the first point, of challenging your brain. After some general advice, we're specifically going to look at brain training: what is it, and does it work? And does it matter how old you are?

Challenge yourself

The aim is simple: challenge your brain with new experiences, as often as you can.

Now perhaps you already do that – you might have a complex, varied job that keeps your brain engaged, or perhaps you have the time and means to travel the world and learn about new places every day. But you might also spend much of your time at home, have a day-to-day life that doesn't hugely challenge you, or simply have other restraints that keep you from doing as much as you used to. Whatever your situation, you should make sure that you are encountering fresh mental challenges every day.

Why challenge yourself?

It's important to continue to challenge yourself, making use of the thinking skills you've built up over the years, so that your brain doesn't start losing the abilities it once had. It's also a good idea to keep on building *new* skills, so that your brain doesn't stop expanding the scope of its learning. As you build new ways of thinking, so you create alternative ways to reach the same conclusion, which can help you compensate for the inevitable effects of ageing.

What challenges should I try?

Given the enormous range of challenging mental activities that you could engage in, you might well wonder which are the most important. But the truth is that there is no one 'right' activity, or set of activities. This doesn't mean that some activities aren't better than others, but simply that there are no specific brain-based activities recommended to the exclusion of all others.

Fundamentally, keeping your brain fit is all about *challenging* yourself. What precisely this means for you will depend on your existing experience, but ideally you want to push yourself outside of your mental comfort zone as much as possible, perhaps by trying a type of puzzle you've never solved, reading a book on a subject you are completely unfamiliar with, or even learning a new language.

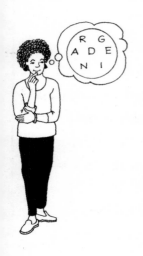

If you want to pick just one thing to start with, learning a new language is an excellent one to try. Even if you never use that language to converse with a native speaker, learning about it will expose you to new ways of thinking, since different languages inevitably encapsulate aspects of the world in different ways. These new ideas can even help enrich your thought processes, since it's easier to consciously think more complex thoughts if you can express them in fewer words – so a wider vocabulary in any language is always likely to be of practical benefit too.

Foreign concepts

The English language includes an incredibly wide range of words, but even so there are concepts that simply can't be expressed by any single English word. You could, however, turn to a foreign language for each of these concepts:

- ► German:

    - *Kummerspeck* – excess weight gained from emotional overeating

    - *Fernweh* – a longing for far-off places

    - *Schadenfreude* – enjoyment of others' misfortunes

- ► French:

    - *Dépaysement* – disorientation in a foreign environment

    - *Flâneur* – an aimless urban stroller

    - *Trouvaille* – something discovered by chance

- ► Spanish:

    - *Sobremesa* – conversation at a table after a meal

    - *Tuerto* – a person who is blind in one eye

- *Merendar* – to eat a snack

► Italian:

  - *Abbiocco* – drowsiness from a big meal

  - *Meriggiare* – to rest in the shade at noon

  - *Ciofeca* – a very badly made drink

► Swedish:

  - *Mysa* – to be engaged in a pleasurable activity

  - *Harkla* – to clear your throat

  - *Fika* – a light mid-morning or mid-afternoon meal

► Dutch:

  - *Uitwaaien* – going out in the wind to clear your thoughts

  - *Afbellen* – cancelling plans by telephone

  - *Gezellig* – cosiness in a home environment

Brain training

You may have heard of the term 'brain training'. It is often used to refer to specific brain games that are said to lead to significant mental benefits.

To be precise, various companies and individuals offer access to services which will provide you with regular brain-training games, and they claim that playing those games will not just make you better at them but will also make you smarter *in general*. This is said to happen via two mechanisms:

1) 'Use it or lose it' – if you don't continue to use your neural circuitry, it will eventually be discarded by the brain; *and*

2) The transfer effect – this is the idea that abilities gained while becoming better at one skill will also 'transfer' to make you better at another. The existence of the transfer effect is generally the justification for any brain training that claims to 'make you smarter'. And it's a great proposition – after all, having a list of specific games which you can play in less than half an hour a day, and yet which provide mental gains that will provide benefit in various unrelated aspects of your life, sounds like the perfect thing for anyone who wants to look after their brain.

But are these claims accurate? We already know that there is potentially some truth in the first claim, as discussed in the previous two chapters, but a key question is then whether these games constitute the *right* sort of mental exercise. The likely answer to this is that, so long as the games continue to vary in a meaningful way, they will indeed be good mental exercise – but if they remain essentially unchanging, or don't change very much, their overall net benefit to you will tail off as you start to become familiar with them. In short, if you're not still improving, you're probably not still learning, and it's time to move on and try something new.

But what about the second, much more powerful claim – that the benefits of the brain games will transfer into other skills, and improve your day-to-day life too?

The transfer effect

Since some key brain training claims rely on the transfer effect, you might wonder how powerful this can be. Well, we do know that such an effect exists at some level, but the truth is that there is considerable debate as to which activities might trigger it, and how powerful its effect might be.

One way to help assess transfer is to distinguish between near and far transfer:

- ▶ Near transfer means that you get better at closely related skills. For example, if you practise a specific memory skill, you might get better at similar (but different) memory tasks.

- ▶ Far transfer means that a seemingly unrelated skill is improved. For example, you might practise an object-packing task in a brain-training game, which would also (via far transfer) improve your ability to solve unrelated logical problems.

As well as considering near versus far transfer, there is also the question of how long an effect might last – after all, if there's only a brief period of benefit, maybe there's no point in training that skill at all.

So is brain training effective?

Brain training is typically assessed on its claims of far transfer, since the most fundamental claim of many brain-training providers is that their games will actually make you generally smarter. Unfortunately, proving far transfer is difficult, and the evidence for it is frequently conflicting. There are plenty of studies that claim to demonstrate it, and then some others that claim the reverse. Independent, overarching meta studies – those studies that combine the results of many studies all together – usually conclude that on balance any claims of far transfer cannot be reliably reproduced. Or, in other words, that brain training does *not* work.

But there's more to this than meets the eye. Firstly, *who* is trying the brain training? It turns out that this is a very important question. And then, secondly, what exactly *is* brain training? Your definition may well affect how effective it is – or isn't. And then there are countless further parameters, such as how frequently you do the brain training and for what session duration, as well as for how many days, weeks or months you follow the programme.

Brain training at different ages

When you were a child, or a young adult, your brain was still developing and learning voraciously. You were also almost certainly exposed to far more varied and novel situations than an older person who is more settled in their routine. You might, therefore, reasonably suspect that following a typical brain-training programme, of limited duration and with only a fixed range of narrow exercises, would not have much effect. It would be unlikely to add up to a measurable improvement in a child's general intelligence – or, in other words, would not show any evidence of far transfer.

The flipside of this observation is the idea that brain training might be of far more reliable benefit to older people than the young. The differing amounts of novelty someone is exposed to in their everyday life will influence the relative gains brought about through brain training. Put more plainly, if you're already being sufficiently challenged, any further challenge may be of negligible effect; but if you are not, then it could be of worthwhile help.

What this all means is that a child learning all day long at school is unlikely to see any significant gain from additional brain-training activities. The brain training will represent only a tiny, narrow part of their learning for the day. Similarly, a young adult making their way through life is already facing large numbers of challenges in their day-to-day life, and those challenges will swamp the complexity inherent in a typical five-minute brain game.

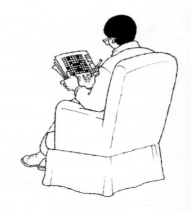

For many people, therefore, it is only as we start to progress through middle age that our lives start to reduce in their level of novel, new-for-today challenges – although, of course, this certainly isn't true for everyone. Perhaps as we approach or enter older age, therefore, brain training will start to have more to offer us. This might also be true of those whose lives slow down at a younger age, perhaps due to having an unchallenging or repetitive job.

Brain-training research

So that's the theory. What happens if we put brain training to the test?

In a six-week study of over 11,000 adult participants aged 18 to 60 following a specific brain-training programme, devised by the UK Medical Research Council, the Alzheimer's Society and the BBC, no significant transfer effect was found – or, in other words, on average those taking part did not have any clearly observable improvement in their reasoning, memory, planning or visuospatial abilities. Brain training did not work.

Why did the brain training fail?

- ► Was it because brain training, in the form used for the trial, just simply doesn't work?

- ► Perhaps the games were too narrow and unchallenging?

- ► Could it be because the people who took part were self-selecting, so they were not typical? It was run online, and those who were curious and motivated enough to sign up to an online test might be the very people who least need the benefits of brain training.

- ► Maybe the 'before' and 'after' tests used to measure improvement simply didn't show up the gains created by the brain training – although these tests were designed to test for the type of gain often claimed for brain training, so this effect should have been minimised.

Given the importance of looking after your brain, it's worth examining this result in more detail.

Brain training complexity

Perhaps the narrow scope of many brain-training games significantly limits their effectiveness. If you're doing the same simple activity over and over, how much benefit would you expect to get?

Brain-training activities often provide practice on very specific skills, sometimes derived from some initial research suggesting that these tasks may lead to general gains beyond merely greater skill at the game itself.

If you practise any brain-training game enough times, you will improve at the game itself, but if that game doesn't reflect a challenge in your everyday life, will it benefit you? If there is no far transfer effect, the answer could be no.

Some commercial brain training involves significant repetition, and yet we know that the brain loves *novelty*. Once it gets good at something, your mental gains from practising that skill are always likely to become smaller and smaller, if the task itself stops changing. It's also likely that small improvements at a specific skill truly are specialised to that skill, and therefore less transferrable.

Another concern is that, if a game becomes repetitive, you may become bored – and a bored brain doesn't tend to learn as well as a more engaged brain. In other words, playing a new brain-training game might well provide you with some initial gain, but over time you would expect any further gains to become smaller and smaller. So your best bet with commercial brain training is probably to try a new programme every so often, rather than stick with the same one for a long period of time, unless it continues to change and evolve. Also, if you find any training to be consistently easy, you can be fairly confident that it is providing almost no benefit at all. Remember, the key point is to be challenged.

n-back brain training

One popular brain-training game is a so-called '*n*-back' activity, where you are asked to alternate between recalling a previous item from *n* steps back in a sequence and learning the next item on a list. So you might be shown a flower and then a car, then asked what object you saw last-but-one – and the answer would be a flower. Next up, you are shown a tree, and asked again what the last-but-one item was – and so on.

Initially, a game like this is a struggle, but with a little bit of practice you soon become much better at it. However, if you then spend a *lot* of time playing a game like this, do you continue to get better? And is this a useful skill in any case? Might you spend a lot of time practising a very specific skill that won't really benefit you? Most of us don't particularly care about getting really good at a brain-training game as an end in itself, beyond any competitive urge: it's the overall benefit we want.

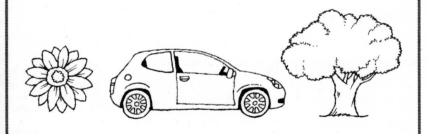

Good brain training

Luckily, not all brain training is created equal. Some well-designed programmes evolve over time to continue to provide new challenges to those taking part. Activities that change and develop over time will provide more mental benefit than those that are essentially set in stone after a certain level of skill has been achieved.

Most studies of brain training have considered only very specific brain-training tasks, and it could be that the problem is more to do with the implementation of the brain-training games in these studies than the actual fundamental concept. That said, a meta study looking for far transfer in those who learned to play either chess or a musical instrument also found that no far transfer took place – but the data was gathered on children, so perhaps the results would have been more encouraging in older adults. It's not really a surprise, as we have seen, that commercial brain training games are of relatively little benefit for children.

Brain training in later life

I've saved the good news for last, which is that brain training *has* been shown to be effective on older people.

A recent study of around 7,000 people found that those over 50, who played a few specific brain-training games for 10 minutes at a time over a period of six months, ended up with improved reasoning and memory skills relative to those who did not. What's more, those over 60 also showed general improvements in their ability to complete ordinary day-to-day activities, improving their so-called quality of life.

Meanwhile, a meta study, summarising a wide range of findings, concluded that far transfer really *does* consistently take place in older adults, What's more, the brain training gains lasted for long enough to be worthwhile – in fact, some memory gains were still effective years after the training had been completed.

In addition to the factors discussed earlier in this chapter, which would suggest that brain training is more likely to be relevant to an older user, it could also be that brain training in older people has a different net effect. It may be that it is more effective in later life because its primary effect is actually to maintain or rebuild existing skills, rather than to actively *expand* your mental horizons. Perhaps its benefit comes not from learning new skills, but simply better maintaining existing ones.

Is brain training worthwhile?

So is brain training worthwhile? Yes – if you're an older adult. For those who are younger, the answer will depend on who you are, and how challenging your everyday life is.

Even if brain training does not provide the mental panacea that is sometimes claimed, it does at the very least provide the chance to practise some specific skills that may be of use – and this is true regardless of whether any transfer effect does or doesn't take place, since the extra exercise for the brain can hardly do any harm.

In fact, brain training may even help the brain maintain existing neural circuitry, so even if you're not getting better, at least you're not getting *worse*. In addition, the sense of achievement the games can bring will help users to feel good about themselves, which is in turn good for their brains.

So my advice is to try a brain-training programme, and see if you enjoy it. If you do, great! If not, don't worry too much – but do make sure that you always take time each day to challenge your brain.

Becoming a super ager

Have you ever wanted to be a super ager? These are the people whose brains carry on working like a much younger person's, right into old age. Most super agers have two things in common:

► They continue to exercise regularly and effectively.

► They continue to challenge themselves with *significant* new mental challenges that regularly take them outside their comfort zone.

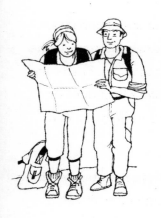

Of course, there are those who do both these things and yet aren't so lucky, but if you want to spin the odds in your favour, these should certainly be two of your primary aims.

How can this book help you with this aim? Well, the exercise part of the equation is somewhat beyond the scope of this book – and plenty has been written about how to look after your body – but the mental challenges part will be well covered. This book is packed full of a hugely varied range of mental challenges.

The challenges in this book come in the form of a really wide selection of puzzles, many of which you may not be familiar with. It might be tempting to skip over the puzzles, or in particular the unfamiliar types – but don't!

As we age, it's much easier to stick to what's familiar, such as a quick crossword puzzle or even a simple word search. But the difficult or unfamiliar ones are in reality the puzzles that are likely to give you the greatest mental benefits. And, when you successfully solve some of these puzzles, the buzz your brain gets will provide exactly the kind of mental reward that will encourage your brain to keep maintaining, and even building, your neural pathways.

Summary

In this chapter we saw just how important it is to keep challenging your brain, and then we looked in some detail at what brain training is and how it might – or might not – benefit you. Ultimately, we concluded that it's a good thing to try in later life, and that there is real evidence that it can be of benefit for people past the age of about 50. At a younger age, its effects may not be quite so important.

In brief

- ► It's important to keep challenging yourself.

- ► Brain training claims to work via the transfer effect, where practising one skill also improves others – but this effect is disputed.

- ► Younger people with stimulating, challenging lives may not see the same benefit of brain training as an older person.

- ► A large study found no significant improvement in the general abilities of adults who tried a specific brain-training programme.

- ► It is possible that some brain-training programmes are too narrow in scope and don't provide a continuing challenge.

► But brain training *has* been proven to lead to significant benefits in older users.

► It is a good idea to look for a wide range of challenges – once a game or puzzle becomes easy, you will gain far less mental benefit from it.

Coming up

In the next chapter, we'll move on from general brain training and start to look specifically at your memory – and how you can make better use of it.

4 Memory

You *are* your memory.

Memory is at the heart of everything: without it, you wouldn't know who you were, where you were, or what you were doing. In a very real sense, therefore, our memories define us.

But what *is* memory? Why do we remember some things and not others? Are our memories trustworthy, and do they ever change over time?

In this chapter, we'll take a closer look at your memory, and find out a bit about how it works. We'll look at the different types of memory, and at how most memories normally don't last – and why that's usually a good thing.

We'll also look at how memories are recalled, and why your memory – particularly for past events – isn't quite as infallible as you might think. We'll explore why some things are easier to remember than others, and look at some memory techniques that can help you better exploit your natural memory abilities.

This chapter also introduces the puzzles and exercises that will be a feature of the remainder of the book. As you are introduced to various memorisation techniques, so there will be a chance to try out these skills right away on the included memory games.

Short-term and long-term memories

Have you ever noticed how you can hear a phone number, or an address, and then can often write it down immediately without trouble? But if you are asked to recall it just a minute later, you might have no idea what it was? If so, that's because it only ever entered your short-term memory. And if you are now wondering what short-term memory is, read on.

First up, it's important to note that *all* learning, from how to walk right through to how to solve nuclear physics equations, can be described as the formation of memories. This suggests that the very notion of 'memory' is incredibly broad. To start to make sense of it, we normally classify memory into three broad classes:

▶ Short-term memory – these are memories that are held in our brains only briefly, and vanish quickly unless we make an effort to remember them for longer;

▶ Long-term memory – these are memories that have lasted beyond the present moment, and which may last for days, months or even years. Memories of conversations, facts and family all count as long-term memory; and

► Procedural memory – these are 'how to do', skill-based memories, which we spontaneously rather than consciously recall. These memories tell us how to run, how to play the piano, or how to make a cup of tea, for example.

So that we can understand a bit more about how memory works, and therefore how we might make better use of it, let's start by looking at each of these three types of memory in more detail.

Short-term memory

Someone tells you their name, and for a brief moment you remember it – but then it is gone. Or perhaps someone reads you their email address, but before you can type it out you realise you remember only the last part and have forgotten the rest. These are both examples of the limitations of short-term memory.

Short-term memory has two key features:

► Firstly, it is just that: short-term, lasting only around 30 seconds or less.

► Secondly, it is very limited. You can't remember a lot of information using it.

More specifically, your brain is capable of holding a few pieces of information in its short-term memory store, all of which will be automatically discarded within around 30 seconds if not consciously repeated or deliberately memorised. The exact amount of information that can be stored varies from person to person, but it is typically around five to seven items.

A short-term memory item, in case you're wondering, is a single 'thing' that you are aiming to remember, such as a word, a digit or a letter. If the items are quite complex, such as a two-part direction ('turn right in 200 metres'), they will probably use up multiple memory slots.

Multiple memories

We have different short-term memory stores for different senses, which means that we can use our short-term memory to remember a greater number of items if they come from multiple senses. This allows you to observe the scent of flowers you are passing, and notice details of the scene you are seeing, while also having a complex conversation. Sadly, it doesn't help you with most things you consciously wish to remember.

Also of relevance is a tighter definition of what makes up a short-term memory 'item'. If, for example, you could somehow compress a long number into a single item, rather than a series of digits, then you would be able to keep more information in your short-term memory. This might also make it easier to subsequently transfer these memories into your long-term memory, should you wish to do so.

Compressing memories

To store more items in your short-term memory, making it easier to remember a greater number of items briefly, you can employ a technique called 'chunking'. It might sound painful, but it isn't – or at least not once you've had a bit of practice!

Chunking refers to combining multiple items into one, therefore increasing the number of things you can store in your short-term memory. For example, given the phone number 305030, remembering it as 'three oh five oh three oh' means remembering six items – but thinking of it as 'thirty fifty thirty' is only three items. In this case, the 'five oh' was chunked into 'fifty'.

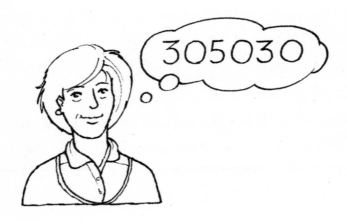

Chunking isn't just a technique for short-term memory – it's a great way of minimising the amount of information you need to transfer into long-term memory too. In fact, compressing memories so that you have fewer separate items to remember is a key part of some memory techniques that we will encounter later.

Working memory

You might also come across the term 'working memory', as a kind-of synonym for 'short-term memory'. Although the definitions are not entirely universal, the difference between the two is usually that short-term memory refers to the ability to recall facts without modifying them in the process, while working memory refers to our ability to work on and modify these items.

For example, if three numbers were read to you and you were then asked to add them up, or repeat them in reverse, you'd use your working memory for that calculation. If you consider how much trickier it is to do mental arithmetic – even simple addition – on numbers you've just heard, rather than merely recall those numbers, it makes sense to distinguish between these abilities. For the purposes of this book, however, we don't need to worry about these differences.

Long-term memory

A long-term memory is, essentially, every memory that isn't a short-term memory. This means, perhaps unintuitively, that anything you remember for more than a minute – and which you aren't simply repeating over and over to keep it in your short-term memory – is in fact a long-term memory. Even if you've forgotten it again just a few minutes later.

Long-term memories are factual stores, such as the name of the capital of France, a family member's birthday, or the plot of your favourite book – as well as what you wore on an important day, how you felt when you met your idol, and what you said when you discovered they were out of milk at the supermarket yesterday.

Multi-sense memories

Long-term memory covers multiple senses, meaning that you might for example recall both the name of a flower and what it smelt like, or both the appearance and feel of a fabric. Research has even shown that, when we recall memories, we trigger the different parts of the brain that previously responded to the original sensations – so to some degree we may literally be re-experiencing the original moment when we recall a vivid memory.

Lasting memories

Long-term memories can last any amount of time, so they might be gone in a day or a week – or it could be months or years.

Memories which we never use do tend to fade away quite quickly, as the brain continues its daily quest to clean up and prune unneeded connections. Conversely, memories which we frequently use, or which the brain attaches significant importance to for other reasons – such as strong emotion at the time of the experience – tend to be more robustly stored.

There are physical changes in the brain associated with the transition from relatively temporary long-term storage (about a couple of weeks) to memories that survive for considerably longer, so it's something that the brain does quite deliberately. Given that it therefore isn't just a question of luck as to what you remember and what you forget, having an understanding of what makes something more memorable is useful when there are things you really don't want to forget. We'll discuss this further, below.

Procedural Memory

Procedural memory is a form of long-term memory, but it's a very specific form connected to actions.

If you ever learned to drive a manual car, you might remember that it seemed at first to be overwhelmingly complex. You needed to balance the clutch with the accelerator, and time your gear changes so that the car didn't suddenly grind to a dangerous halt. But then, after a few hours of practice, it started to get easier.

With this practice, you no longer needed to consciously think about exactly what your feet were doing, and could concentrate more on coordinating your multiple actions. And then, with further practice, the entire act of changing gear started to become subconscious, and you found you could shift gear without thinking anything more complex than 'I want to shift gear'.

Eventually, you probably found yourself changing gear without even consciously noticing you were doing so. Indeed, once driving lost its novelty, you might even have sometimes found yourself in the somewhat disconcerting situation of realising you had driven a familiar route without consciously noticing much of the process.

How did you gain these new, innate driving abilities? Well, it was all thanks to your procedural memory. This is the part of your brain which learns to perform common tasks without your conscious attention, so that you don't need to concentrate on the move mundane parts of life.

Untangling procedural memories

Procedural memories often become so automatic that, although you know exactly how to do something, you may lose the ability to actually *explain* what you are doing. In other words, you are able to perform the overall action but cannot describe the individual movements that it involves!

For example, while most drivers could explain how to change gear clearly enough, what about how to ride a bicycle? How exactly *do* you shift your weight around to balance the tendency of the bike to fall to the left or right? And what is the method you use for deciding how much to lean into a corner so that the outward forces don't tip you over? The chances are you would struggle to put any of these bicycle-riding explanations into words, certainly with any level of detail.

The truth is, when you first learned to ride a bicycle, you consciously leaned to one side or the other as you went, but after a bit (or a lot) of practice this became entirely automatic – so automatic, in fact, that most of the time you are oblivious to the fact that you are doing it, and you therefore end up having no idea of what *exactly* you are doing. You just do it. And that's all thanks to your procedural memory.

Memory loss

Forgetfulness is good! No, really. In fact, forgetting things from your long-term memory is one of nature's major survival mechanisms.

There are very rare historical examples of people who had great trouble forgetting anything, and their lives were very difficult as a result. Just imagine, say, if you could remember every shopping list you'd ever had. It would be incredibly confusing each time you went to the shops. Now expand that to all aspects of your life, and you'll probably be immediately thankful as to just *how* forgetful your brain really is.

Filtering the world

The ability to filter out what's unimportant, and remember only what remains, is critical to enjoying life. If you recalled every fact you'd ever heard, you'd be overwhelmed with information – and, apart from the ability to win *Mastermind*, this would be of little practical benefit to you.

The act of forgetting is the process of refining what's important – and what's not. Being able to instantly recall only the most relevant information about something is incredibly helpful, since it prevents you being unable to see the wood for the trees. You can then always use those initial memories to rack your brain for additional information, or use them as the basis for further research online or in a library.

Do we forget skills?

When we forget things, these are rarely from our procedural memories. This means that physical skills we acquire tend to stay learned – so once you are able to play the piano, or to juggle, you'll always have a basic ability to do those things.

Consider: do you know anyone who completely forgot how to drive, or how to ride a bike? Such forgetting would usually be the result of a mental illness, since these memories are not normally discarded. If you went a long time without using them, it might take some practice to get up to speed, but you'd be unlikely to completely forget them. This is lucky, since it would be annoying to have to learn to drive again if we spent a year or two without a car!

Day-to-day memories

At this very moment you can almost certainly recall, at least after a little effort, exactly what you've had to eat today. But if you were asked tomorrow about today, would you still be so certain? And what about the day after? Or next week?

Most day-to-day memories are stored temporarily, but, when we turn out not to need them, they soon fade. They also get lost in a sea of very similar memories on subsequent days. So, since individual meals typically aren't particularly remarkable, what we eat isn't usually that memorable.

Conversely, if you have something very special to eat, or it is combined with an enjoyable social occasion, this may elevate it far beyond a normal day-to-day memory. For example, I still remember arbitrary details of the moment I discovered I liked pizza, such as where I was sitting and in what room. Not very useful, truth be told, but clearly, that pizza-eating event had a marked impact on me! Similarly, you in turn might remember a meal many years later, if it was on an important date or a special occasion. Or involved pizza.

Now you might not particularly care that you don't remember what you ate for very long, but understanding *why* you don't remember it is useful. Ultimately, most day-to-day memories will fade away, and the less novel and unusual the memory is, the faster it will fade. This is why you might recall parts of a conversation with a friend you rarely see even a year later, but have already forgotten what someone you see every day said to you just a day ago.

Distant memories

Many aspects of our memory fade with time, no matter how well we might have once remembered them. Moments that once seemed unforgettable do tend to soften, and even if we revisit them from time to time, this doesn't mean that they won't fade at all. What's more, the less well we remember something, the more prone it is to being altered.

Remembering an individual fact, such as Paris being the capital of France, is a fairly binary thing – you either remember it, or you don't. Once you know it, you might well remember it for the rest of your life without trouble. But our personal memories are far more complex, since each thing we think of as a single memory is really built from a large number of smaller, discrete memories that are then gathered all together. So, while we might remember aspects of days from long ago, we slowly lose certain details over time.

Changing your memory

Have you ever changed your mind about a decision? Of course you have. But did you know you have almost certainly also changed your *memory* about things too?

Not convinced? Well, that's not a surprise – we don't realise it's happening.

We think of our memories as being like miniature documentaries that we can replay at will, but the truth is more complex:

> ▶ Firstly, we can remember only what we observe, and if our observations were inaccurate for some reason, the initial memory can be very misleading. Perhaps we misheard someone, or didn't see somebody standing behind a pillar and so completely misinterpreted a situation. Or maybe we came upon a situation halfway through and misunderstood what we saw. Whatever the reason, when we later come to retrieve the memory we

forget the haziness and remember what we *think* we observed.

▶ Secondly, no matter how observant we were, we don't remember *every* detail of an event. Our brains therefore have to reconstruct the event each time we recall it. Essentially, what happens is that we retrieve as much information as we can from our memory, and then – just as happened originally with our perception of what was happening – we piece together the scene from these memories. We interpret it again, even if we don't realise we are doing so.

The overall effect of the imperfection of our memory is that we can be quite convinced of things that are completely untrue, and yet not be deliberately lying to ourselves.

We've already seen how revisiting a memory is key to reinforcing it, but if we don't retrieve it accurately, we can also *modify* it – so each time we misremember what happened, we can become ever more convinced of our actually incorrect recollection. Plus, as we start to forget aspects of the memory, a 'cat's whispers' effect can take place, where the memory of the event starts to modify itself in ways of which we are completely unaware.

Manipulating your memory

Your memories aren't as fixed as you might think, but when you privately recall an event any changes are typically accidental.

But did you know that people can deliberately attempt to change your memory – without you even realising it?

In the previous section, we mentioned how memories of events are reconstructed from lots of individual memories. This is a powerful technique used by our brains, since it means we can store just the key facts and then reinterpret the event each time we recall it, avoiding remembering lots of unnecessary details. But it has a major weakness. *Because* the memory is reconstructed from individual memories, the corruption of just one of those memories, or the insertion of a false memory, means that they can then become part of a convincing – but completely false – narrative, which we nonetheless truly believe is our own, unmanipulated memory.

Leading questions

Memory changes can be triggered by something as simple as being asked a question that *presupposes* something that never happened. For example, if you witnessed a traffic accident and were asked whether the collision location was 'before or after the pedestrian crossing', you might later recall a pedestrian crossing as part of the scene, even if such a thing did not exist. Your brain immediately forms a mental image from the description to try and answer the question, but may also unwittingly insert it into your actual memories of the event. The question cannot be answered, but in your attempt to do so you may convince your brain of a falsehood.

91

Disney's Bugs Bunny

In one study, a third of volunteers became convinced that they had seen Bugs Bunny at Disney World, despite the improbability of this -- since Bugs Bunny is not a Disney character. This happened simply by virtue of them being shown a fake advert where Bugs Bunny greeted people at Disney World, and being asked if they remembered meeting him there too.

An even greater percentage were convinced of the false memory if they were first primed by the placement of a large cardboard cut-out of Bugs Bunny in a waiting room.

What this, and other similar studies, suggest is that anyone who claims to be able to recover 'long-lost' memories should be treated with caution. Our memories are easily influenced by the exact phrasing of a question, or other material, and some people can be easily led – whether intentionally or not – into recalling things that never actually happened.

Fallible memories

Let's look at memory weaknesses in a bit more detail, since most of us think of our memories as fairly infallible – if we firmly believe we have remembered an event correctly, we are unlikely to doubt ourselves. It can therefore be hard to understand just how vague many of our memories really are.

We might, as an example, think we remember conversations word for word, but research has shown that in reality (unless we are specifically learning lines) we remember concepts and how they go together – so we remember the gist of what was said, but not the exact words. This, of course, is problematic, since it means we remember *our* understanding of what was said, which could be completely wrong if we misheard a key word, or misconstrued some body language.

Misheard words

It's not just our eyes that can deceive us. Similar processes happen for our hearing too – we stitch together the *most likely* thing we are hearing from various cues, including:

- ► the actual acoustic sounds we hear;

- ► where in space we think they are coming from;

- ► the lip movements we can see;

- ► and, to a significant extent, the things we actually *expect* to hear, based on the speaker, context and so on.

How often have you guessed at a word in a conversation on the basis that it seemed by far the most plausible option? Well, this happens unconsciously for every single word, for varying degrees of uncertainty. Now, imagine recreating a scene from your imperfect, fragmented memories of an already imperfectly observed situation. Is it any surprise that they may not be the perfect recording we expect?

Our memories are also fragmented, as mentioned, so when we think we recall something in detail, we are in practice stitching it back together from many parts into what seems the most likely form.

Even right now, your brain is making many informed guesses about the world around you in order to make sense of the vast amount of information arriving at your eyes, ears and other senses. This is why you don't need to puzzle out the shape of each letter in this paragraph – and also why you might sometimes see a face on the surface of the moon, even though your rational mind tells you it isn't really there.

Memory loss with age

We've seen how our memories can fade with time, as well as become less reliable. And, in previous chapters, we have seen how memory loss is additionally naturally associated with ageing, and that memories become slower to store and retrieve as we grow older.

This combination of naturally fading memories, along with age-related changes to our memory, can sometimes lead us to think that our memory is a lot worse than it really is. We've been forgetting things our whole lives, but as we age we have far *more* things to forget since we have experienced more, so it's only natural that we will come across more and more situations where we realise we no longer recall something as well as we believe we once did.

Severe memory loss

We are all different, so some people will have much more noticeable memory loss than others as they age. But how do we know if we should start to worry?

The truth is that a level of memory loss which might be a natural effect of ageing in one person could be an indicator of something more serious in another, so expert advice is always required in diagnosing any problems.

One warning sign, however, is a loss of procedural memories, manifesting perhaps as trouble remembering how to cook a common meal, to get dressed, or even how to get to the supermarket to buy food.

Another warning sign is forgetting seemingly unforgettable information, such as your own name or a loved one's name. But unwittingly using the wrong name from time to time is a common mistake, and not usually of concern unless it starts to be the rule rather than the exception.

If you are concerned about yourself or a loved one, raise these concerns with a healthcare professional as soon as possible. Some brain illnesses can be paused or controlled, if they are treated early.

If you do find yourself having more trouble remembering day-to-day events as you age, you can try to counteract this by making an effort to pay greater conscious attention to what's going on around you than you are used to having to do. For example, make an effort to maintain clearer focus on conversations, and more consciously take note of things you want to be sure to remember – for example, by repeating them back to yourself.

What makes something memorable?

Memory loss is a double-edged sword. There are things we *want* to remember, but also sometimes things we *want* to forget. So how does our brain know which is which?

Memorable moments

Our brain looks for indicators that something is important to us. Moments of high emotion are one such indicator, which is why you may recall many details of where you were or what you were doing when you heard about major historical tragedies such as the *Challenger* disaster, or the 9/11 attacks. The same is often true of other moments of high drama too, such as the first moon landing. Of course, it might not actually be useful to remember these details, but to your brain they were moments of great importance.

We don't want to have to manufacture moments of high drama in order to remember things, however, so what can we do instead? Humour is one option – things that are funny or remarkable in some way trigger feelings that make them intrinsically more memorable. The use of humour – or deliberately ridiculous images and associations – therefore forms part of various memorisation techniques, where whimsical connections between objects are used to make them easier to remember.

Rhythmic recall

Creating rhymes can help make things more memorable. This works even if the rhymes don't seem particularly helpful. For example, generations of children were taught that, 'In fourteen hundred and ninety-two, Columbus sailed the ocean blue'. The number rhyme doesn't seem like it should help, since countless numbers end in 'two', and yet it really can work.

Pay attention, and rehearse

Fundamentally, remembering something is about *paying attention*. We need to be properly focused. It's also about *rehearsal*, so we reinforce the memory.

What's more, if we really want to remember something, we should ideally expose ourselves to the same concepts in different ways – so we *really* pay attention, and rehearse it in different ways to cover the same information from different angles. Some memory techniques to help with doing this include:

► taking notes, so you are forcing yourself to consciously focus on each point;

► explaining a concept out loud to ourselves (or others), so we are engaging an additional part of our brain; *and*

► writing and then answering questions on a subject, so you present and interpret it in a different form.

These methods all force us to pay attention, and to cause different parts of our brain to handle the same information.

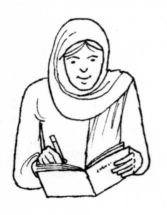

This helps us to strengthen the associated memories.

Rehearsal certainly also helps. You could try revising the information you wish to memorise in an hour, a day, a week or even a month later, depending, of course, on how long you wish to remember it for.

Losing your keys

Have you ever put your keys down – or your glasses, wallet, purse, or similar – and then forgotten where they are?

We've all done it, unless you have somewhere specific where you always place these, and are disciplined enough to always do so.

We forget where we put our day-to-day belongings because we aren't paying attention, which in turn helps to demonstrate just how important attention is to the formation of memories. The reason for this is the mundanity of the action – it's something we do every day, putting down our keys when we enter our house, so it just doesn't seem that important to our brains.

If you don't want to lose these objects, make sure you specifically say to yourself where you have put them when you place them down – then at least you have a chance of being able to retrieve that memory, without having to mentally 'walk back' through what you did to guess at where you might have put them. Or, of course, you could simply make sure you always put them down in the same place.

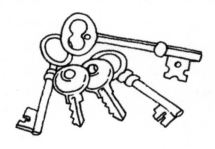

Memory retrieval

Memories are often retrieved via associations, meaning that we remember something closely connected to the memory we actually want, and then use that to jump across to the memory we actually need. It's one reason why, the more we know about a subject, the easier it becomes to learn more on it – much easier, perhaps, than when we knew relatively little about the subject. It therefore follows that *deliberately* linking memories to existing knowledge can be really helpful.

Linking memories together, via associations between them, can help minimise the number of times that we feel sure the memory is there, but we just can't manage to retrieve it. The 'tip of the tongue' effect (discussed in the next chapter, pages 136–7) is a similar effect.

This also suggests another good method to help memorise something, which is to look for a way to connect it to something you already know about. Not only does this help us reinforce the memory, but it also provides an additional way to retrieve that memory from our brains.

Linked retrieval

Association between memories is the reason you might, for example, hear a song and immediately think of when you first heard it; or answer 'Paris' to a quiz question and find yourself thinking of a trip you once took to France. Associations also

Linking memories

The best way to build associated memories is to learn more about a subject, but it can also be used as a memory technique when you need a shorthand method to help learn something.

Let's say that you know that the moon landings were known as the 'Apollo' programme, but you want to remember that it was Apollo *11* that first landed mankind on the moon. To help with this, you could try visualising the '1's as rockets, so you can always find a connection to the mission number once you start to think about the Apollo rockets.

This might seem a somewhat ridiculous connection, but ridiculous connections can be memorable, and any connection is better than no connection – plus, it gives an example of how abstractly you can think if you wish.

Another worthwhile linking technique is to try and learn reverse connections too – so as well as remembering that 'a' connects to 'b', you also try to connect 'b' back to 'a'.

follow on from one another, so once your French trip comes back to mind, you might find yourself thinking of places you visited there, who you were with, what time of year it was, and so on.

Conversely, associations can sometimes be *unhelpful*. For example, if you have a good friend called Jim, and then at some point meet someone else called Jim, your brain is tempted to assume that some of the characteristics of your friend apply to this new person – even though that is completely illogical. Similar responses can also lead to discriminatory beliefs, whereby people may not even consciously realise they are profiling people based on race or other attributes. Sometimes it's important to challenge ourselves, and to try to understand exactly where our beliefs and gut instincts are coming from.

Memorisation techniques

We've touched briefly on some ways to make things memorable, which can be summarised as:

- ▶ Pay attention

- ▶ Rehearse

- ▶ Repeat the same information in different ways

- ▶ Use humour if appropriate

- ▶ Link memories to one another.

Now let's look at some more practical examples of how we can use techniques based on these general observations to improve our day-to-day memories.

Historical memorisation

Nowadays we are used to writing everything down, and with the advent of modern technology, it has become even easier to do so – and also easier to access any information we might want to retrieve. But for most of history this has been far from the case, and different memorisation techniques have been invented over the years. Some of these are for general use, while others are most appropriate for specific situations.

In a preliterate age, memorisation techniques were taught to children from an early age. People grew up using them to remember both their family history and their folklore, as well as more day-to-day matters. Their memories were not intrinsically better, but they would have been highly practised at remembering things efficiently.

Nowadays, we rarely need to make much conscious use of our memory, once our schooldays are behind us. Most people store contacts, birthdays, appointments and more in either electronic or written form. On a mobile phone, these are available to us instantly, no matter where we are. We write down shopping lists, and we can search online for the answer to almost any question we might have (or, at least, *an* answer). We don't even have to remember the day and time of our favourite TV show, either.

Day-to-day memory practice

Since we don't *need* to remember day-to-day things, why should we make the effort to do so?

One answer is that, as you age, it's important to make greater conscious use of your memory. This doesn't mean you shouldn't write things down, particularly if they are important, but whenever it is sensible to do so, try to remember them *as well*, such as the time and date of an appointment, or even directions to get to a particular location.

You can also try using memory exercises, such as writing down sets of digits, words or names and then seeing how many you can memorise. Or you could find a set of facts you've always fancied knowing – such as the names of all the countries in Africa, or the appearance of every flag of the world, or even the dates of the reigns of every English monarch – and set about learning them. This might not be of any immediate, direct use (unless you are entering a quiz championship, perhaps), but the exercise is good for your brain.

A small selection of memory exercises is included on the following pages, but these are just a taster to get you started. You should make an effort to consciously use your memory whenever you can.

Remembering names and faces

Have you ever been introduced to someone, then just a few moments later realised you've forgotten their name? Some people seem to have a preternatural ability for it, but many of us struggle with remembering names.

Remembering names and faces gets harder as you age, although, if you've found it hard your entire life, you might not have noticed! The secret, ultimately, is to concentrate. If someone tells you their name and you simply say hello without making any particular effort to remember it, the chances are that you won't.

These are two key steps in forming a lasting memory:

► The first step is to repeat the name back to yourself. Repetition helps memories form, and the act of consciously repeating it forces your attention.

► Secondly, you want to associate the name with the person, since associations help you retrieve memories.

Repeating a name back is fairly self-explanatory, but how do you go about linking a person with their name?

Linking names and faces

There are various methods you can use to link a face to a name, and which will be most relevant will depend on who the person is and how it is that you know them. If, for example, this person is a bank manager and you are unlikely to forget that particular fact, you could try linking their name to their job, but in most cases, it is easiest to link their name to their appearance. Their appearance will therefore be the method you use to trigger the memory, and so specifically you want to find some sort of connection – preferably a memorable one – from their appearance to their name.

Linking a name is tricky the first few times you try it, but like many things, it gets easier with practice. The first thing you can try is to think about what characterises their appearance. Maybe they have bright blue eyes, or perhaps they walk with a limp, have pitch-black hair, or wear exaggerated glasses. Whatever it is, try to find an amusing or rhyming way to link it to their name, since – as we've seen – these characteristics intrinsically make something more memorable.

Alliteration can work really well, perhaps because it combines a natural rhythm with something that might be amusing. For example, a Bonnie with blue eyes could be Bonnie Blue, or a David with strange glasses could be David Double-eyes. That might sound offensive, but these memory aids are private just to you. You probably shouldn't tell anyone about the nicknames you create for them!

By the time you have thought about their name enough to come up with your connection, you have already done a great job of paying attention to their name, and effectively rehearsed it several times. This, along with the connection you have created, will make it much easier to recall their name in future. Then, take a moment a bit later in the day to go over the connection in your head, and you'll reinforce it further.

Try it now
There's no need to wait until your next social occasion to try out this technique!

Take a look at the six people on the page opposite, and the names associated with them. Spend as long as you think you need to memorise the name that goes with each face. Then cover up the top illustration and see if you can attach the correct name to each face. (Also, bear in mind that these faces have very few clear features, so if you manage it with these images then you might find it even easier with real people!)

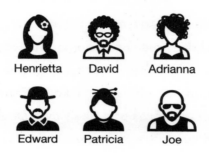

Now cover the pictures above. Can you write the name of each person under their picture?

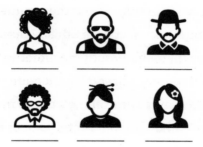

How did you do? If you couldn't remember them all, does it help to know that the first letter of the six peoples' names are A, D, E, H, J and P? Initial letters can help prompt your memory.

Connecting objects

The memory technique for remembering faces, described above, is based on finding memorable connections. But what if it isn't names that you struggle with, but everything else? Well, a similar technique can also be used to remember lists of objects, plus, it can be useful for memorising them in a particular order, should you need to do so.

Instead of linking a face to a name, you now link any arbitrary pair of items, and then keep on linking them together into a long chain. So long as each link is memorable, you can then follow the links and retrieve all of the items you connected together. It might sound a bit unlikely, but it really does work – and it isn't as much effort as you might imagine!

Say, for example, that you want to remember bread, milk, orange juice and broccoli. To make them memorable, you want to link them together in unusual ways – and the easiest way to do this is by making strange, visual connections. These should be so unusual that they will be inherently memorable. For example, you might imagine a loaf of **bread** that is being used to stir a huge vat of <u>milk</u>; the milk bizarrely starts to turn into **orange juice** as it is stirred; and then out of the orange juice start to sprout florets of <u>broccoli</u>. Sounds bizarre? That's the point.

Using a method like this, you can turn mundane objects into a sequence that is considerably easier to remember. You then only need to remember the first word – which was bread, in the example above – to trigger the connected memories of the other items.

Why does this work?

This technique works for all the same reasons it works for faces:

- ▶ it forces you to pay attention;

- ▶ it encourages you to rehearse what you want to remember; *and*

- ▶ it provides strong associations to help you retrieve the memories.

As noted above, you do still need to remember the first object – but you could always link it to something else that would trigger it. This is a shopping list, so if you can find a way to link 'shopping list' to bread – such as by imagining it being written on the side of a loaf of bread – then you can help recall the first item just by remembering that you *have* a shopping list.

Visual connections

Vivid visual connections are often easier to remember than those that are more abstract and harder to picture in our heads. This might not be surprising if you consider, for example, that you can probably successfully identify many photographs or pictures that you have seen before, even when shown them again many years later – your visual memory is remarkably powerful. Forming visual connections also requires additional parts of your brain to get involved, which may intrinsically make you pay better attention.

Visual numbers

For objects that are harder to visualise, you can try representing them in other ways. Numbers in particular don't have a readily available visual image.

In some cases you can work around this. If you need five bananas, for example, you could try imagining them in the shape of the Roman numeral 'V'; or if you need two pounds of sugar, you could imagine a pair of boxing gloves (for pounding) hanging from the bag of sugar. But these are imperfect solutions.

More advanced memory techniques involve sitting down and learning a strong image to associate with every number from at least 0 to 9 – you can then always construct longer numbers by linking these together. Or, better still, by learning a separate image for every number you are likely to need.

This might sound like a lot of work, but it only needs to be done once. Then, in the future, if you wanted to remember that, say, your friend lived at Number 35, and you knew that 35 was represented by a dancing giraffe (because, why not?), then you would simply think of your friend dancing with a giraffe – and you'd probably never forget that they lived at Number 35.

Try it now

You won't need to remember any numbers for the following exercise. Simply spend as long as you like studying the image below, making note of which objects you can see in it. Then, turn the page and see if you can spot which objects are missing.

As a hint, you could try starting with one of the items and then building connections to other items in turn. For example, perhaps the <u>bike</u> is riding along on the <u>skates</u>, which get stuck on a <u>leaf</u>, which is then cut in half by the <u>shears</u>, which cut the <u>plants</u>, which grow into <u>pencils</u> that are placed like fingers into the <u>gloves</u>, and so on and so on.

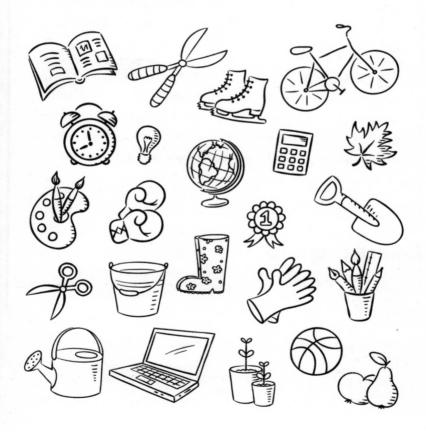

Now take a look at the following arrangement. Some objects have moved, while others have vanished. Can you list all of the items that are missing?

How did you do? If you think you missed some items, why not turn back the page and try again for the remaining objects? You'll know if you've remembered them all if you recalled eight objects that are no longer there.

Remembering facts

Do you know the order of the planets, heading out from the sun? Or the order of successions of the Tudor monarchs?

Sometimes we want to remember specific sets or sequences, such as those listed above. In these cases, one potential memorisation method is to create your own abbreviations, acronyms or acrostics. You then use these to prompt you with the initial letters of the set or sequence.

Memory – in brief!

Abbreviations, acronyms and acrostics work best when:

▶ **you know the items in a set, but want to remember their order; *or***

▶ **you have trouble remembering the items in a set, but are likely to recall them if prompted by their initial letters.**

Acronyms

The acronym technique involves packing lots of information into smaller pieces. It's therefore a chunking method, as discussed earlier in this chapter, pages 80–1.

To see how to create an acronym for memorisation purposes, consider that the order of colours in a rainbow is red, orange, yellow, green, blue, indigo and violet. This can be remembered in acronym form as ROYGBIV, or perhaps more imaginatively as a name, Roy G. Biv. Both of these are just about pronounceable, so can be used to remember the seven colours of the rainbow, as well as their order. You just need to learn one seven-letter word (or name), and hey presto!

This works as a memory technique because we already know the colours, and can retrieve them when prompted by the initials. Orderings are fairly abstract concepts, so it's much easier to remember an acronym than to remember an explicit ordering such as 'red is next to orange; orange is next to yellow; yellow is next to green' and so on.

You can also use acronyms to help remind you of the items in a set. As an example, I once needed to learn the names of the four bases in DNA for an exam. To do so, I simply memorised the fun-sounding acronym G-CAT, and – at the time – that was all I needed to be able to recall that they were guanine, cytosine, adenine and thymine. It really did work in the exam, too.

Abbreviations

Abbreviations are essentially acronyms where you relax the rules, so they are another chunking technique.

Perhaps you want to remember that the Tudor monarchs were, in order, Henry VII, Henry VIII, Edward VI, Mary I and Elizabeth I. This gives you the initial letters of H, H, E, M and E. There are two different Es, however, so you might want to abbreviate these to Ed and El, or maybe Ed and Liz – or you might decide you definitely know Elizabeth I was the last of them and just the two Es is fine. Also, perhaps H should be He, and M should be

Ma, so they are easier to pronounce? If so, this could give you HeHeEdMaLiz.

Now that might not be particularly memorable in this form, so you could experiment until you find a form that you personally find more memorable – such as by adding spaces so it reads 'He heeds ma, Liz!' Notice that I've added in an 's' to 'Ed' so it makes a bit more sense, and is therefore easier to remember.

This might all seem a lot of effort for memorising five names, but remember that you need to do it *only once*. From then on, this information will be ready to hand – once you've learned your abbreviation!

Acrostics

Depending on the subject matter, and how much you need to learn, acronyms and abbreviations might not always be the best choice. You can't always form a useful abbreviation, no matter how hard you try.

In these situations, another method to try is to use an acrostic, which is where the first letters of each word spell out a useful sequence of initial letters. For example, a traditional phrase for remembering the order of the rainbow is 'Richard of York gave battle in vain', since the initial letters correspond to the colours in order. As another example, you could help yourself remember the first five elements of the periodic table – hydrogen, helium, lithium, beryllium and boron – by memorising 'Help him learn both bits'.

Making your own acrostics can take some practice, and it can be tricky if you have a lot of words that start with relative rare letters. But, since it's your own private memory aid, you can use whatever rules you like. You might, for example, decide that words of three or fewer letters are always to be ignored when using your acrostics. Then you'd have no trouble adding in various prepositions, conjunctions and other linking words to help structure a more memorable phrase.

Other techniques

If you struggle making your own acronyms, abbreviations or acrostics, a much more general method for learning sequences is simply to try breaking them up into separate facts, memorised one at a time. For example, given the colours of the rainbow, you could learn that red is followed by orange, and then once you are happy that you know this and can reliably remember it, only then do you go on and learn that orange is followed by yellow. And so on.

Another, even more general, method for learning facts is to broaden your knowledge of a subject. If, for example, you want to remember the names of the Tudor kings of England, it will help if you know something about them. The more facts you have at

your disposal, the more your memories can form associations
to help you retrieve the information you want. If you read more
widely on the subject, returning to the relatively basic fact of their
ordering will make it seem (and it will actually *be*) easier to learn.

Learn when you're at your best

Most people find that they learn better at certain times of day,
rather than others. When you have the flexibility to choose a
time of learning, experiment to see when works best for you.

If you're not sure where to begin, try the afternoon. Various
studies have suggested this works best for many people.

Try it now

See if you can learn each of the following sets of facts. You can
spend as long as you like on each set – not just minutes but even
days, if you wish.

You could use any of the techniques discussed so far, as you
prefer – or even a technique of your own. Then, when you are
done, see if you can recall the sequences without referring back
to this book.

▶ **The planets in decreasing order of size**

Can you memorise this ordering of the planets in
decreasing size, starting with Jupiter and working down
to Mercury? Note that this list also includes a numeric

value for the relative size of each planet, but these are just for interest and there's no need to learn these figures (unless you want to!).

1. Jupiter – 1,120 per cent the size of Earth

2. Saturn – 945 per cent the size of Earth

3. Uranus – 400 per cent the size of Earth

4. Neptune – 388 per cent the size of Earth

5. Earth – 100 per cent the size of Earth (of course!)

6. Venus – 95 per cent the size of Earth

7. Mars – 53 per cent the size of Earth

8. Mercury – 38 per cent the size of Earth

▶ **The first 10 US presidents**

Can you learn this list of the first 10 US presidents? The notes of the years in office for each president are just for interest, but since they are either four- or eight-year terms (with one exception), they shouldn't be too tricky to learn – should you wish to.

1. George Washington, 1789–97

2. John Adams, 1797–1801

3. Thomas Jefferson, 1801–9

4. James Madison, 1809–17

5. James Monroe, 1817–25

6. John Quincy Adams, 1825–29

7. Andrew Jackson, 1829–37

8. Martin Van Buren, 1837–41

9. William Henry Harrison, 1841 (died in office)

10. John Tyler, 1841–45

▶ **Geological eras, from most recent to most ancient**

This geological set could be tricky to learn since the names of the eras, particularly the more ancient ones, may not be familiar – but if you look closely, you'll spot that there is considerable repetition of prefixes and suffixes, which should help. Even if you don't manage to learn them all, it will still be a good challenge to try.

There's no need to learn the associated time periods – they are just for interest.

1. Cenozoic: 66 million years ago to present

2. Mesozoic: 252 to 66 million years ago

3. Palaeozoic: 541 to 252 million years ago

4. Neoproterozoic: 1,000 to 541 million years ago

5. Mesoproterozoic: 1,600 to 1,000 million years ago

6. Palaeoproterozoic: 2,500 to 1,600 million years ago

7. Neoarchean: 2,800 to 2,500 million years ago

8. Mesoarchean: 3,200 to 2,800 million years ago

9. Palaeoarchean: 3,600 to 3,200 million years ago

10. Eoarchean: 4,000 to 3,600 million years ago

How did you do with the sequences? If you've successfully recalled them, congratulations! Now make a note to try them again tomorrow – and again next week, or the week after. Will you still remember them then?

Memory palaces

In the 'Connecting Objects' section on pages 107–112, we mentioned that you could use an image for each number in order to make it easier to remember quantities, but that this would require you to pre-learn these images.

Another technique that requires some initial learning is the 'memory palace' method, but the exact amount of learning will depend on how many items you wish to be able to remember. For just a few objects, relatively little learning is required, and it is such a powerful technique that it is well worth taking the time to do so.

What is a memory palace?

The basic idea behind a memory palace is that you imagine a journey through a location or series of locations familiar to you, and then use these as places to associate with objects that you wish to remember. By learning the journey once, you can use it over and over again to both store and retrieve objects in order.

This journey might be through your house, or some other building you know well – or even multiple buildings. Once you've imagined your journey, you memorise it. You only need to do this once, and then forever more you will be able to use it as your memory palace.

Using a memory palace

To use your palace to memorise something, imagine progressing through your learned journey. As you enter each room, you associate the next item that you wish to memorise with that room, in as memorable a way as you can. You then carry on entering rooms, memorising items, until you have learned everything you want to remember. Of course, your memory palace needs to be extensive enough to cope with the number of items you need to learn.

When the time comes to recall the items, you simply stroll back through your palace and see what you've 'stored' in each room. So long as your association links are strong – in the ways we've discussed already – this technique allows for very rapid recall because, by reusing the same route over and over, you don't need to waste time trying to remember the trigger items. They're always the same.

An example palace

Let's say that your memory palace journey involves entering your hall, going into your living room, moving on to the kitchen, going up the stairs, and then entering a bedroom.

You start by imagining that you are entering the first room in your memory palace journey, and look around for a way to connect the first object to that room. For this to work, it's important that you have chosen locations familiar to you and which you can visualise.

Say, for example, that you want to remember to buy writing paper, a birthday card, apples, some cakes and stamps. Here's one potential way that you could remember these example objects in the example palace:

- In your <u>hall</u>, you wallpaper the walls with the <u>writing paper</u> you want to buy;

- you enter the <u>living room</u> and are surprised to see an enormous <u>birthday card</u> filling the entire room;

- as you go into the <u>kitchen</u> you notice that the taps have been replaced by apples, and <u>apple juice</u> flows when they are turned on;

▶ the tops of the bannisters on the <u>stairs</u> have been replaced by small <u>cakes</u>; *and*

▶ the duvet on the bed in the <u>bedroom</u> has been replaced by one made out of thousands of postage <u>stamps</u>.

Now, when you want to recall the sequence of objects, you imagine walking through your memory palace. The strong, visual associations created by you make it easy to remember what you placed in each room. In fact, even though the story above was not your own memory palace and not your own associations, you might well be able to remember all five objects just by being prompted by the route: hall, living room, kitchen, stairs, bedroom.

Extending your palace

After building an initial small memory palace to see whether the technique works for you, you can expand it over time by adding further rooms – so long as you stick to ones that you can visualise. Maybe your house now links across to another location, or perhaps you simply visit more specific locations in your house – the cupboard under the stairs, the cabinet in the bedroom, the wardrobe in the bedroom, and so on. You could even add exotic locations, such as a swimming pool, bowling alley, island beach and so on.

Another way to expand a memory palace is not to visit rooms, per se, but rather to visit objects in the house. So you might start at a coatrack in the hall, move to a pinboard, then head to the sofa in the living room, the TV in the living room, and so on. You might even find this an easier method, since it can be simpler to connect items to specific objects rather than an entire room. It's also relatively straightforward to add objects into your memory palace, when you need to expand it, particularly if they correspond with real-life items that are familiar to you.

Try it now
Pick six rooms familiar to you, and write their names here:

_____   _____   _____

_____   _____   _____

These will represent your memory palace for now, on the assumption that you haven't yet memorised a route. If you have, you can use that instead of writing some rooms above.

Now use a journey through those six rooms to remember the following set of items:

1) Broom

2) Wig

3) Cat

4) Newspaper

5) Marshmallows

6) Handbag

Then, once you are ready, see if you can recall them on a blank piece of paper. Transfer the list of six rooms first, to represent what would normally be your pre-learned memory palace route.

Next, make a note to try recalling the items again tomorrow. Can you still remember all six items? You might well be able to, so long as you are prompted by your memory palace journey again.

You could also try writing out your own lists of items, and seeing if you can use the memory palace technique to memorise and then recall these too.

Summary

In this chapter we've looked at your memory in detail, and seen how it works and how we can make better use of it.

We started by considering how your short-term memory is both limited and brief, and how lasting memories need to be transferred into long-term memory by paying attention to them. These memories can then be strengthened by repetition. We also saw how procedural memories allow us to learn to perform physical skills without much conscious thought.

Long-term memories fade, so we discussed how and why this happens, and saw how *some* memory loss can be a good thing so that we don't get overwhelmed with useless information. We saw how your memories of events are reconstructed from lots of smaller memories, and the problems that can stem from this, including how these memories may not always be as accurate as we imagine. We also saw how memories can be altered, deliberately or otherwise.

Next, we looked at memory loss with ageing, and considered why some things are much more memorable than others. We considered emotions, rhythm and other memory techniques, including how we can deliberately create links between memories in order to make them simpler to retrieve.

We went into detail on some particular memory techniques:

► Remembering names and faces.

► Connecting objects with visually memorable links.

► Acronyms, abbreviations and acrostics for remembering sets and sequences.

► Memory palaces – a powerful general technique for remembering lists.

We also tried some memory exercises, with a particular focus on trying out the specific memory techniques we described.

In brief

► Memory is central to everything we are.

► Memory can be classified into short-term memory, long-term memory and procedural memory.

- Short-term memory is forgotten after 30 seconds, and has limited capacity.

- Chunking is one technique for keeping more in your short-term memory.

- Long-term memories may be remembered for varying lengths of time.

- Procedural memories are skills we gain which don't require conscious attention.

- Memory loss is important for managing what we store.

- Day-to-day memories fade unless they are somehow special.

- Memories can be unwittingly modified.

- Memories are not literal recordings, but involve guesswork when being reassembled.

- Ageing can make some normal memory-loss issues seem much worse.

- Moments of high emotion are very memorable.

- Humour, rhymes and alliteration are also memorable.

- We have to pay attention to remember.

- Repetition helps us strengthen memories.

- Building strong associations makes memories easier to recall.

- Amusing connections from faces to names make people easier to remember . . .

- . . . and amusing connections in general help associate memories, making them easier to recall.

- Visual schemes for numbers can be learned to make them easier to memorise.

- Acronyms and abbreviations are chunking techniques that are useful for learning facts.

- Acrostics are another memory technique for memorising ordered lists.

- Broadening your knowledge on a subject can make it more memorable.

- Time of day can affect learning ability.

- The memory palace technique is a powerful way of learning lists of items.

Coming up

In the next chapter, we'll move on to look at memory in a much more general sense by considering how important it is to engage in lifelong learning.

5 Lifelong Learning

How much do you think you have learned this past month?

However much it was, the chances are that – from your brain's point of view – it wasn't enough!

It's time to put that right, by making sure you challenge your brain every day.

Continuing to challenge your brain throughout your life is one of the key steps you can take to help preserve your existing mental abilities heading on into later life, as well as to help build new ones.

We've already seen how unused brain circuits may be dismantled, and rarely used memories will eventually be discarded. Not only this, but the natural effects of ageing are also responsible for the loss of brain cells, requiring additional effort simply to maintain the status quo. With changes like this, it might seem that resistance is futile – but that's not the case at all. It turns out that looking after your brain is a key part of a healthy and rewarding life.

Ensuring that your brain continues to learn throughout your entire life should be as important a part of your daily routine as making sure you stay as physically fit and healthy as you can, if not more so. And when it comes to learning, the more challenging the content, the better – so long as you can understand it well enough not to lose interest, at any rate.

Expanding horizons

A great aim is to try to expand your horizons in some way, by trying something new. New experiences are inherently challenging, and therefore help improve the richness of your thoughts and build multiple ways of reaching the same conclusion.

Are there things you always wanted to do, but which you never tried? Perhaps you now finally have the means or the time to do them. Or you could consider taking up other new activities, which you have never previously even thought about – or which perhaps didn't even exist some years back. The more out of your comfort zones these activities take you, the better, so long as it doesn't involve inappropriate risk.

Controlling time

You can even slow time – or at least your own perception of it – with experiences that are far from your norm.

Don't believe me? It's true. When you do something that is completely new to you in some way, and become completely engaged in that activity, the richness of the experience is likely to cause your perception of time to slow down. For example, I once spent a week on a snorkelling trip to various reefs, having never tried it before, and that week felt like a fortnight or more – quite the opposite of the usual holiday feeling where it seems that the entire trip has passed in a flash. And that's the flipside of it too – if you spend a week happily 'doing nothing', it really *does* seem to pass quickly, since your brain isn't stimulated in the same way.

You might recall that even relatively short periods of time seemed to last *forever* when you were a child – a 20-minute journey appeared to take what would now account for hours, while an extended school holiday period felt almost unbounded in length. This was because much more of the world was fresh and new to you as a kid, so your brain was learning at a much more rapid pace. Your perception of time was therefore very different.

In life and death situations, people sometimes describe time as almost appearing to stop, and becoming hyperaware of everything happening all around them. But you don't need to put yourself in danger to experience this same effect – although so-called 'adrenaline junkies' actually do precisely that, paragliding off tall buildings and surfing waves 15 metres

(50 feet) high. Luckily, just doing something completely new can be enough, so long as you find it exciting and engaging.

Time and ageing

As we age, it's natural to find that time seems to pass more quickly. Partially this is because we have been alive longer and so have a different perception of relatively shorter periods of time, but it's also because our brains are less challenged. The way to work around this is simply to ensure we don't just sit back and let time pass us by. If you feel that every day is passing in a flash, you may not be challenging yourself sufficiently – although, of course, it's also important to sometimes take a break, and rest, from time to time. Being in tune with the requirements of your body becomes even more important in later life.

Challenge yourself

Expanding your horizons need not require travel to exotic locations. At the simpler end, you could learn a new word each day, perhaps from any of the various online 'word of the day' services, or simply by flicking through a paper dictionary. Or you could read an introductory guide to a subject you know little about – whether that's particle physics or reading the entertainment news, or how to play bridge or train a horse, or

even something incredibly esoteric, such as the history
of the potato.

Another option is to take up a new hobby involving physical
movement, whether that's learning to juggle or do magic
tricks, how to paint watercolours or even how to cook in a new
style of cuisine. Or, if you are able, you could visit new places –
this need not be far, and could simply be to visit shops you've
never previously been into, or to drive a route you've never
tried before. Anything that is new in some way is better than
the alternative.

Travel, if an option for you, is a great experience for your
brain – so long as it's to places that are new to you. Revisiting
the same places over and over will not bring the same benefits.
Different cultures have different conventions and norms, as
well as different styles of architecture, different types of food,
and so on – plenty of things to interest and challenge our
brains. Some of this will happen subconsciously, but making
an effort to look around and observe your surroundings is a
great idea. Combining this with learning (or simply trying
to get by in) an unfamiliar language adds even more
mental benefit.

If you can't travel far, you could try looking *up*. In many towns
and cities, raising your eyes above the level of the street can
reveal all kinds of hidden history and architecture – many places

look very different when viewed above street level. Or you could look for details you would normally ignore – researching the history of a site or town, for example – and seeing if you can spot the results of this history in the physical locations.

Take up new social activities too, if you are able. Social interaction is very important for your brain. Even if you find it difficult, you should still try – without it, you really aren't doing all you can to look after your brain. This need not be too strenuous – it could be as simple as talking to your neighbours, or chatting to people at a church group. Better still, join a club or society and take part. You can look in local newspapers or magazines for ideas, or the local council might have a list of nearby organisations. You could even take adult education evening classes. Other options are to volunteer to help with a charity, or other institution. These activities will all involve new challenges, adding extra benefits for your brain over and above the social interaction itself.

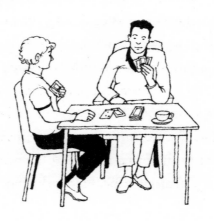

It's tempting in later life to rest on your laurels, but if you wish to maintain everything you've worked for, it's important to keep the mental pace up, or even increase it, if appropriate – even if your physical pace might slow down at some point.

Words and language

Without language skills, how do you think conscious thoughts? There is some evidence that full consciousness can arise only once our language skills have developed, so challenging yourself with word puzzles is a great way of keeping these critical skills in good working order. Forming cogent sentences and thoughts also makes use of your short-term memory, while recalling words and concepts makes use of your long-term memory.

Simply extending your vocabulary can be of benefit. Being able to represent your thoughts in fewer words, which becomes easier as your vocabulary expands, increases the complexity of the concepts you can contain in your short-term memory and so may effectively make you smarter. Some people, such as serious Scrabble™ players, can take this to extremes where they learn considerable quantities of words without knowing what they mean – but it's a far better brain-training activity to learn words along with their meanings. The richer your understanding of a word, the better. So, next time you come across an unknown word in a book or crossword puzzle, look that word up and find out more, even if you already have the gist of the meaning.

What's more, this extra information and attention also helps make the word easier to remember.

The 'tip of the tongue' effect

Have you ever tried to remember a word but found yourself unable to recall it? In those situations, are you sometimes sure that you know the first letter of the word but just can't remember the rest? If so, you're not alone. The 'tip of the tongue' effect is a well-known psychological phenomenon, and it reveals something very interesting about how your brain works.

Manual filing systems often index contents by the first letter of a name, and it seems this is how the system works inside your head too. It turns out that your brain recalls a word based on the first letter, so if the retrieval of the word gets stuck at that stage, you can find yourself being fairly sure of just the initial letter, but unable to remember the word itself. Sometimes with a bit of effort you can then recall the complete word, but in the meantime you often feel a strange angst while you strain to find it. So long as you don't have this effect so frequently that it interferes with your day-to-day life, it's nothing to worry about – it's just a feature of how your brain works.

'Tip of the tongue' tips

Next time you have trouble recalling a word, don't agonise over it – make a written note if it's important, but then try to forget about it. You could, for example, change the subject if you were talking, or make a conscious effort to think about something else. Later on, you might find that you can suddenly remember it, unprompted – after all, your brain is remarkably good at carrying on thinking about things without your conscious effort.

You can also try using the 'tip of the tongue' effect to your benefit. If you can't think of a word at all, see if you can instead try to recall just the first letter. If you're correct, which you might well be, this can then sometimes help you recall the desired word. Or if you can't think of the first letter, work through the alphabet in your head, trying each letter in turn. You can try this out with the anagrams in the following section, by experimenting with starting the word with each letter in turn.

Vocabulary puzzles

The following puzzles are all about word recall, and will make you think in various ways.

Try not to skip over the puzzles you find the trickiest – these might well provide the most benefit. Conversely, don't be afraid to take a break and come back to a puzzle later, if you are having trouble with it.

A to Z

The aim of this puzzle is a relatively simple one. All you need to do is place a different letter of the alphabet in each empty square, so that you end up with a valid crossword grid. This means that you should be able to read an English word in every across and down run of white squares, once complete.

Letters along the sides of the grid are provided for you to cross off and keep track of which letters you've already placed. Note that there may be multiple ways of completing some words, but there is only one way which allows all 26 letters to be placed once each.

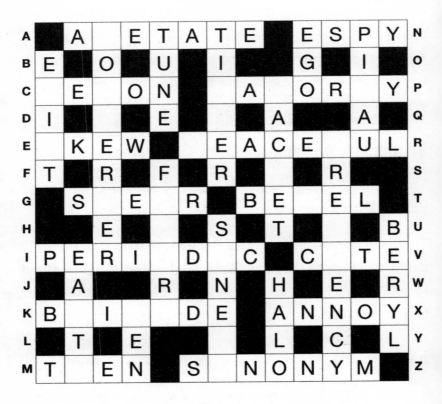

Zigzag

This puzzle requires you to use your vocabulary skills to write letters into the empty, grey squares so that each row contains a complete word. The last two letters of each line must also form the first two letters of the following line, as indicated by the grey stripes.

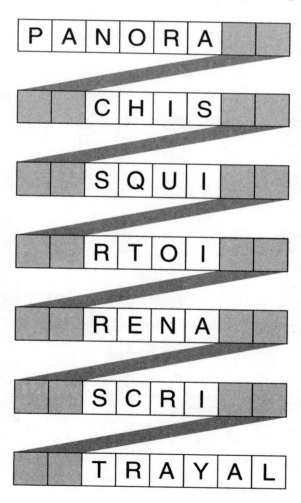

Anagrams

Each of the following lines contains an anagram of a mammal. Can you rearrange each set of letters to reveal them all?

If you get stuck, try using the 'tip of the tongue' effect to your advantage by experimenting with starting the word with each different letter found in the anagram.

Another useful hint is to try writing out each set of letters in a circle or in a random 'letter cloud' – changing the visual ordering of the letters in this way can help your brain see new possibilities for arranging the letters.

1. THE PANEL
2. NEAT POLE
3. FIG FEAR
4. RICH SOONER
5. TENT AREA

How did you fare with the anagrams of mammals? If you solved a few or more of them, try this set of longer anagrams – these are all of countries.

1. KIND DIM TONGUE
2. AS A RITUAL
3. BAD BOARS
4. IN A GLOOM
5. FAN AS HATING

First and last

In this next puzzle, you can practise running through the alphabet to help you find a word. Specifically, in each of the following entries the first and last letter of the word are missing, *but* they must be the same letter. For example, _GEND_ is missing an 'A', to make AGENDA.

If you get stuck, try working your way through from A to Z until you find the answer – and if you miss finding it, try again more slowly. Perhaps the word is not pronounced the way you would expect, after the missing letters are added.

1. _AUSTI_

2. _TUDIO_

3. _OCA_

4. _AI_

5. _RI_

6. _IDO_

7. _ULOGIS_

8. _RIM_

9. _ARO_

10. _OA_

Letter sequences

One type of vocabulary puzzle that can be unexpectedly tricky is the letter sequence, as might be demonstrated by the puzzles below!

The aim is to work out what each set of initials is short for. For example, M T W T F would represent the days of the week: Monday, Tuesday, Wednesday, Thursday and Friday. Can you identify all of the following sequences?

1. J F M A M J J A S O N D
2. R O Y G B I V
3. O T T F F S S E N T
4. M V E M J S U N
5. T F S S M T W
6. H T Q F S S E N T
7. K P C O F G S
8. H H L B B C N O F N

Initial letters

Can you identify each of the following novels and their authors from just the initial letters of their titles and names?

1. TKAM by HL

2. TGG by FSF

3. MD by VW

4. BNW by AH

5. TPOMJB by MS

And how about these films?

1. GWTW

2. TSOM

3. BCATSK

4. OFOTCN

5. CEOTTK

Now try these Shakespeare plays:

1. RAJ

2. JC

3. KL

4. AYLI

5. MAAN

And finally, these famous works of art and their creators:

1. ML by LDV

2. TSN by VVG

3. GWAPE by JV

4. G by PP

5. TPOM by SD

Word circle

How many words of three or more letters can you make from the letters in this word circle? Each word should use the centre letter plus two or more other letters.

Each puzzle includes one word that uses *all* of the letters.

In this first puzzle, see if you can find 20 words; a total of 35 or more is excellent.

1

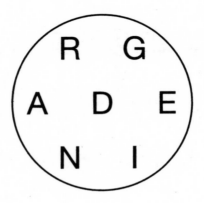

Now try this second word circle, which has a greater number of letters. Once again, 20 words is a good target, while 35 words or more is excellent.

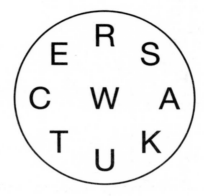

Word square

Words can sometimes be easier to recall in a more constrained situation. In each of the following word squares, see how many words you can find by starting on any letter and then tracing a path to neighbouring letters. The path must travel only horizontally or vertically between letters, and shouldn't revisit the same square within a word. Each puzzle contains one word that uses *all* of the letters.

1

C	O	L
A	R	E
T	E	S

Targets: Good = 15 words;
Excellent = 25 words

2

T	R	R	A
H	O	P	I
I	W	E	S
N	E	S	S

Targets: Good = 15 words;
Excellent = 25 words

Deleted vowels

It can often be easier to think of the words we want when restricted to a particular theme, such as the names of classical composers or safari animals.

In this puzzle, all of the vowels have been deleted from a set of five flowers. Can you restore the vowels and reveal the original words?

1. DFFDL

2. BTTRCP

3. GRNM

4. RCHD

5. FCHS

Now try this set in which all of the vowels have been removed from a set of five European capitals.

1. LNDN

2. PRS

3. MSCW

4. THNS

5. SL

Every other letter

This puzzle is similar to the previous one, but now every other letter has been deleted from each word. How quickly can you restore the missing letters to reveal the original words?

First, can you find five musical instruments?

1. V_O_I_

2. _U_T_R

3. U_U_E_E

4. _I_N_

5. C_A_I_E_

And secondly, can you find five types of fruit?

1. O_A_G_

2. _I_E_P_L_

3. B_A_K_E_R_

4. _E_T_R_N_

5. P_A_H

Word prefixes

This puzzle is another test of your vocabulary skills. Each of these five words is missing its initial **prefix**. Can you attach the correct prefix to the correct word, to form a new word? Each prefix and each word is used only once.

Prefix	Word
Anti	action
Inter	amble
Post	climactic
Pre	impose
Super	modern

Word suffixes

Now try this similar task involving word suffixes. Can you attach each suffix to the correct word, so that each suffix and each word are used once to make five new words?

Word	Suffix
Abstract	ful
Catch	ous
Numb	ment
Cavern	our
Wish	ness

Word fragments

Some words have been broken up into pieces and then mixed together. Can you reassemble them to reveal the names of five occupations?

1

ARD	ARMA	CIAN	CIST	EGU
ELEC	IAN	ICI	ISTI	LIF
PH	SOL	STAT	TOR	TRIC

Now try reassembling the names of five cocktails:

2

COSM	DA	GAR	HAT	IQU
IRI	ITA	ITAN	JI	MAN
MAR	MO	OPOL	TAN	TO

Hidden words

This is a different type of vocabulary puzzle that can sometimes prove surprisingly tricky, given its relative simplicity, and which involves embedded hidden words.

Each of the following phrases or sentences includes a hidden colour, split among the letters of multiple words. Can you find them all? As an example, the phrase 'Mea<u>gre en</u>ergy' contains the hidden colour 'green'.

1. When in the woods I yell, owls hoot.

2. He often looks for angels.

3. Can you spin knives quickly?

4. I pluck just one eyebrow now.

5. I want a better education!

Now can you find a hidden number in each of the following?

1. On bank holidays he won't work.

2. Easter is an occasion English people may celebrate.

3. We stuff ourselves on Christmas Day.

4. Nothing can outweigh the joy of summer.

5. New Year's Eve nicely bids goodbye to December.

Codeword

In the more advanced vocabulary puzzle overleaf, the aim is to write a letter in every empty square so that each across and down entry is filled with a regular English word – just like a completed crossword grid.

Each letter is associated with a number from 1 to 26, and it's up to you to work out which letter has which value – although some are given for you, to get you started.

Solving the puzzle will initially involve some experimentation to try out various possible fits for letters. To narrow down the options, look out both for very frequent letters and for those that appear as double letters. The last few letters in a word can sometimes be quite revealing, too.

Use the squares beneath the grid to keep track of which letter has which value, and keep track of which letters you've already assigned by using the letters on the left and right of the grid.

	N/O/P...												
A	14	18	22	22	6	23	■	22	11	4	10	16	19
B	10	■	19	■	18 **R**	■	9	■	9	■	25	■	15
C	6 **P**	21	19	18	22	25	13	24	10	■	8	13	18
D	10	■	10	■	25	■	1	■	21	■	22	■	22
E	25	22	18	■	22	1	10	18	19	15	18	22	5
F	14	■	■	■	12	■	18	■	■	16	■	25	
G	■	12	6	10	25	14	■	19	10	6	10	10	■
H	13	■	18	■	■	26	■	9	■	■	3		
I	7 **G**	18	10	23	15	22	12	25	14	■	10	21	19
J	25	■	16	■	21	■	13	■	10	■	17	■	18
K	22	5	10	■	13	25	19	10	18	8	21	16	10
L	18	■	14	■	20	■	10	■	9	■	16	■	21
M	10	23	10	8	12	9	■	3	23	3	19	10	2

Right-side labels (top to bottom): N, O, P, Q, R, S, T, U, V, W, X, Y, Z

1	2	3	4	5	6	7	8	9	10	11	12	13
14	15	16	17	18	19	20	21	22	23	24	25	26

Language Puzzles

Many word puzzles involve solving clues that point to particular words. In this next set of puzzles, you will be using clues to help you find the correct words.

Word pyramid

One type of clue-based puzzle is a word pyramid, in which each row of the pyramid uses the same set of letters as the previous row, but with one extra addition. The letters on each row are not necessarily in the same order as on the previous row, however.

Because the rows are interlinked, you can help your brain retrieve possible words by considering the letters you are given. Trying out different possible first letters of words can sometimes help, as can looking for potential prefixes or suffixes that might account for some of the letters.

See if you can solve the clues to complete each of these word pyramids:

1

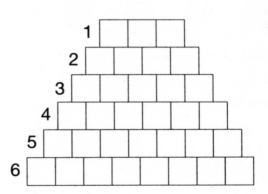

1. Part of a curve
2. Feel concern
3. Strongly desire
4. Cuts into slices
5. Certain winter garments
6. Fissure

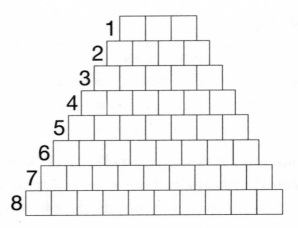

1. Fruit with a tough shell
2. Metre, gram or pound
3. Join together
4. Unit of time
5. Certain sonata movements
6. Transport route end
7. Thinks deeply about
8. Small replica models

Crossword

The 'tip of the tongue' effect (see also pages 136–7) can be seen when solving word puzzles too.

If you've ever solved a crossword, you'll know how useful it is to reveal the first letter of a word by solving a crossing clue. Indeed, the first letter of a word often helps more than even a few other letters in the same word. This is why crosswords are generally easier if you start at the top and left, and aim to fill down and to the right – and why if you find these first clues tricky, you'll often find the entire puzzle tricky even if the later clues aren't so hard.

Crossword grid designs vary, and the most fiendish ones are designed so that you get far fewer first letters to help you. Next time you encounter a crossword grid, check the top row and leftmost column of a grid – if they contain one or two words that fill most of the width or height of the puzzle, it's probably going to be easier to solve than if you only have lots of 'uncrossed' starts of words at the edges of the grid.

You can try out this theory with the crossword overleaf:

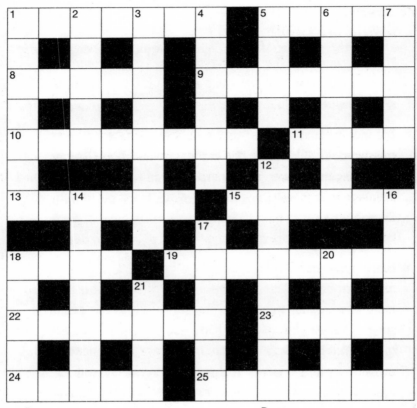

Across

1 Microchip element (7)
5 Decorate; embellish (5)
8 Many times (5)
9 Runner or jumper, eg (7)
10 Inclination (8)
13 Fermenting agents (6)
18 Noisy seabird (4)
19 Committee president (8)
22 Branch of mathematics (7)
23 Sydney suburb with a famous beach (5)
24 Figure of speech (5)

Down

1 In a moment (7)
2 Ancient Roman language (5)
3 Coloured paper scraps (8)
4 Subtlety (6)
5 Dull throbbing (4)
6 Aromatic culinary herb (7)
7 Nephew's sister (5)
12 Dependable (8)
14 At a brisk speed, in music (7)
16 Real (7)
18 Allow, as in a request (5)
20 Fervour (5)
21 Competent (4)

Cryptic crosswords

The crossword on page 156 is a 'straight' – also known as 'quick' – crossword, meaning that all of the clues are simple synonyms or other direct clues.

The trickier counterpart to this type of crossword is the 'cryptic' crossword, in which every clue includes some indirect, cryptic way of defining the answer. These puzzles can appear like another language to those who are unfamiliar with them, but in truth it doesn't take a long time to learn how to solve them, at least at a basic level – there are only a small range of common clue types.

Every cryptic clue includes both a straight definition, as in a regular crossword (although these are allowed to be trickier and more obscure than in a normal puzzle), plus a cryptic definition – so you are given two ways to solve each clue, if you are able to work out how to split the clue into its two components. Very occasionally all the words in a clue work simultaneously as both a definition *and* a cryptic clue, but this is unusual – although it can be very impressive, when successfully pulled off.

What sometimes makes cryptic puzzles appear more complex, however, is that they can rely on conventions which have amassed over many years, so some clues can seem completely intractable if you are not 'in the know'. A classic example is the phrase 'on board', which for historical reasons is usually permitted to clue the letters 'SS', as an abbreviation for 'steamship' – and for those letters to be wrapped around other letters, as if they were 'on board' the steamship. Ignoring odd esoteric complexities such as this, however, cryptic crosswords are nowhere near as complex as they can appear to the uninitiated. And, just like almost any other type of puzzle, they can vary from easy through to extremely hard.

If you've never tried cryptic crosswords, or only dipped a toe in the water, it is well worth taking the time to learn more about them. They are great mental workouts, requiring all kinds of clever thinking to solve. In many respects they are the ultimate word puzzle, with a huge variety of mental gymnastics needed to tackle them successfully.

Word play

These puzzles include a different type of word play, where various well-known idioms are represented in a visual way. Can you work out what each image represents?

1

violet violet violet violet

2

THROUGH THROUGH

3

0 it it

4

5

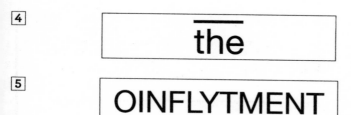

Summary

In this chapter we looked at how important it is to continue to challenge yourself every day, and to make a genuine effort to do so by pushing yourself out of your comfort zone. We saw how your perception of time changes depending on the novelty of the experience, and how this can help counteract the feeling of time passing too quickly as we age.

We looked at various possible ways you can start to introduce more challenge into your life, whether by reading more widely, taking up new hobbies or engaging in more social interaction. We also saw how travelling to new places – or just trying to experience existing places in new ways – can be of help.

Next, we considered our language skills, and how critical they are for our conscious thought. We saw how extending our vocabulary is of benefit to us, and considered what the 'tip of the tongue' effect tells us about how our memories are retrieved.

Finally, we looked at lots of different vocabulary and language puzzles, all of which provide excellent, varied challenges for you to try. As part of this, we also considered why cryptic crosswords are the ultimate word puzzle workout, and well worth investing the time in learning to solve.

In brief

- ► Challenging yourself through life is key for your brain.

- ► Try expanding your horizons with new activities.

- ► Really novel experiences can slow your perception of time.

- ► Expanding your horizons can start at home.

- ► Regular social interaction is really important for your brain.

- ► It's a good idea to continue trying to expand your vocabulary.

- ► The 'tip of the tongue' effect can be used to help remember words.

- ► Solving a variety of word and language puzzles is one way to challenge yourself.

- ► Cryptic crosswords are a great mental workout.

Coming up

In the next chapter, we'll look at the importance of a positive outlook on life, and consider some of the things you can do to help ensure you stay cheery.

6 Staying Positive

Have you ever found yourself complaining about something, and then realised you don't really have a reason to be upset? It can be quite easy to find fault in things, and much simpler to criticise than to make constructive comments.

As we get older, it's tempting to compare many things unfavourably to 'how things used to be'. But the truth is that our memories of the past are not the accurate portraits we think them to be, as we've seen in the previous chapters. Our recollections of events become progressively less representative, so it's very hard – if not impossible – for us to objectively compare the current day with a long ago past.

In this chapter, we'll look at how important it is for your brain that you have an upbeat attitude to life, even in times of adversity, and so we'll consider some ways to help make you feel better – and look at why this might get easier with age. Next, we'll look at the placebo effect, and see what it tells us about how our brains sometimes jump to incorrect conclusions. We'll also look at self-confidence, and ways to deal with mistakes and regrets.

Happy and positive

Would you rather be happy or sad? Sometimes sad things happen over which we have no control, but almost all of us would surely say that we would rather be happy, given the choice.

And what about being positive? Positivity is generally associated with happiness, so it's almost always the case that positive people are happier than negative people. And therefore, in turn, it's not hard to see that – since we all want to be happy – it's worth trying to be a fairly positive person.

Being happy and positive makes you feel good, but did you know that there's an even more important reason to try to be happy and positive? Well, there is: it's really important for your mental health too.

A happy brain

We learn best when we are happy and relaxed. Perhaps this makes intuitive sense, since when we are unhappy or stressed it can be harder to focus and pay attention in the way that we've seen is necessary to form lasting memories. That said, small amounts of stress can *help* us focus, by putting enough mental pressure on us that we start to get things done.

It's not just about focusing, however, since varying emotions cause our brains to behave differently in all kinds of ways. These changes are usually temporary, except if the emotions start to last for a very long time – weeks, for example. Being in a perpetually sad or stressed state is not good for you, and it will start to affect your mental abilities in ways that can become permanent, if left untreated. It can also affect your physical health too, since your brain controls the rest of your body.

Helping your brain

If we stay in a particular state for too long, our brains start to adjust to it as the 'new normal'. If that state isn't a great one, that's not a good thing. So what can we do about it?

▶ Physical exercise – particularly vigorous exercise – is a great way to cheer yourself up, even if in a less happy state it can sometimes seem too much trouble to bother. And yet, once you start significant aerobic activity, your body starts releasing feel-good chemicals into your bloodstream. These pick-me-ups, known as endorphins, work to cheer you up. You also start to feel good about yourself for actually doing the exercise, so you get a double whammy of happy feelings.

▶ Laughter really *is* a good medicine for some ailments – so, when you are feeling glum, try watching a recording of a comedian you enjoy, or reading a book that you know can make you smile.

► Another method that works for a great many people is simply to listen to music – preferably music that you know you enjoy, so you can relax as you listen to it. Music can have a transformative effect, lifting you out of the moment and invoking different feelings that help distract your brain from its previous state. (In fact, if you've ever tried watching a film without its musical soundtrack, you'll realise just how important the presence of music is for creating mood!)

► Social contact can also be a great way to cheer ourselves up, even if the conversation itself isn't that exciting. The need to come 'out' of our own heads, and interact with other people, naturally helps our mood to shift. This can at the very least 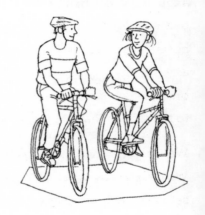 help to start the journey back towards a more positive mindset. (Social contact has other benefits too, but we'll discuss those in a later chapter.)

Age gives you perspective

The good news is that, as we age, research has shown that we tend to have a naturally more positive outlook on life. Or, at the very least, it becomes easier to see the positive side of an experience.

This might be because we have seen more of life, so we can put events into better perspective than we could when we were younger. It might also be because we tend to feel less of the angst and uncertainty of youth, with some aspects of our lives perhaps less up in the air than they once were. It could also be because our cerebral cortex has better learned how to deal with any unhelpful interventions from the more basic parts of our brain, which sometimes responds in simpler, less nuanced ways to the things that happen to us.

We also become better able to spot the upside in situations. With more life experience, it's easier to see how even a potential setback can perhaps be informative for the future, which encourages a more glass half full attitude to life.

The placebo effect

One of the most astonishing demonstrations of the power of positive thought is the placebo effect. This is where a person has a perceived benefit from a medical treatment, when in fact the medical treatment itself did not bring about that benefit.

Medical mysteries

Time and again, people feel the expected effects of medical treatments, even when those treatments have not actually had that effect at all. This outcome, known as the placebo effect, is a huge problem in medicine. When given sugar pills rather than medicine for relatively minor ailments, many people report the same results as those taking the medicine – so long as they believe they have had the medicine, not the placebo.

This effect is so powerful that it can be very hard to test some medicines. Sometimes medicines that were once thought to work well have been discovered to have no direct effect, with their only benefits coming through the placebo effect. It is particularly difficult to separate out this effect when assessing drugs for complex mental conditions, such as depression, where – for some patients, but certainly not all – a firm belief that they are getting better can form part of the healing process.

People feel better because they expect to, so powerful is our brain's ability to be influenced by positive thinking. And while

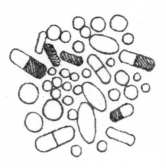

positive thought may well make us *feel* better, it can actually also help us to *get* better too, because – as we have seen earlier – when we are sad or unhappy for a long period of time, our brain and body start behaving differently, and in a way that is not conducive to good health. Sadly, however, no amount of positive thought can heal a serious disease on its own.

One of the most interesting things about the placebo effect is that it demonstrates just how important and beneficial it is to maintain a generally positive attitude on life, and how it really does help keep you healthy.

Alternative medicine: what is it?

Some people swear by alternative medicines. An alternative medicine is essentially any treatment used for medicinal purposes which isn't recommended by mainstream healthcare providers, due to a lack of scientific evidence for its claimed medicinal effect.

Alternative medicines run the gamut from herbal medicines through to other treatments that are chemically equivalent to sugar pills. In almost all cases, their effectiveness comes from the placebo effect, which can for some people be reinforced by a religious belief in the power of the treatment.

When used as treatment for less serious conditions, such as a cold or some other illness that will eventually go away of its own accord anyway, these substances can be helpful because they encourage a positive attitude. A negative outlook really can discourage healing, as we have seen. And, what's more, after taking medicine you believe to be effective, you may start to feel some of your symptoms less acutely, as your brain handles the information it's receiving in a different way.

Risks of alternative medicine

The downside of alternative medicine is when people believe it to be something that it is not.

Alternative medicines cannot cure serious health issues, since positive thinking cannot do so, and positive thinking is all they provide. It's therefore important to understand that these treatments, if chosen, must be combined with other techniques that have been proven to work. There have been reported cases where patients have delayed treatment of cancer by trying alternative therapies first and later come to regret this decision.

Think of it this way: for century after century, humanity tried countless medical techniques that, in the case of serious diseases, all failed. It was only when modern medicine started to develop that we actually started to be able to heal ourselves in a reliable way. And yet alternative medicine therapists may claim that the same ancient herbal medicines or other techniques which failed for millennia are now suddenly just as effective as modern medicine. Well, history proves this to be very unlikely.

We want to believe

Alternative medicine also provides an insight into the fallibilities of our brains when it comes to experiencing the world around us.

Using the example of cancer again, some people who start chemotherapy find that the treatment is so unpleasant they feel unable to finish the recommended course and turn instead to alternative treatments. By that point, the initial part of the course may have dealt with the immediate cancer, but – as the side effects of the chemotherapy start to subside – they go on to believe that the alternative medicine they switched to is responsible both for their apparent improvement over the following weeks and the removal of the cancer. Their brains falsely link the alternative medicine to the result, and they become convinced that it was successful for them. Unfortunately, since a full course of chemotherapy treatment helps reduce the chances of recurrence, people who prematurely turn to alternative medicine are more likely to become sick again – all because of the tendency of our brains to misunderstand cause and effect.

Self-confidence

We've seen that age tends to make us feel more positive. But does it also make us feel more self-confident too?

Age gives us experience, so we become better able to judge our own knowledge against that of others. This therefore means that we should naturally become more self-confident, since we are more secure in our own beliefs and learning. There may even be specific tasks – such as speaking in public – that no longer bother us in the same way they once did.

Even so, there is often a surprising difference between the level of self-confidence of those who, through experience and knowledge, deserve to feel self-confident, and those who really don't. It's worthwhile, therefore, taking the time to realise just how self-confident you really *should* be.

The ignorance of others

It's easy for someone else to feel confident when they are unaware of their own ignorance, and indeed it is a strange truth that less-informed people generally feel far more confident than better-informed ones. Our brains have evolved in such a way that we often have an instinctive response, or a 'gut feeling', about things – probably so that we could make rapid decisions when the need arose – but in many cases our instinctive behaviour involves simplification and the avoidance of detail. Perhaps this is why we often have no trouble blindly accepting viewpoints that don't stand up to serious inspection.

Put another way, it's easy to believe you are knowledgeable on a subject when you lack the knowledge to know what you *don't* know. It's typically only as you start to gain expertise on a subject that you begin to realise just how extensive your ignorance is. Paradoxically, therefore, the more you learn about a subject, the *less* confident you might become.

Remembering the wins

There is a tendency in many sizeable organisations for the most reckless – or clueless – people to rise to the top. This is particularly common in large financial institutions, for many decisions in such industries are tantamount to bets on what is likely to happen. Those who are most ignorant or most reckless often make the most unwise, largest bets – and, although they may often lose them, they will also inevitably 'win' some of them. If they win enough, people acclaim them as visionary leaders, forgetting their bad decisions. Anyone who raises past failures after a major success is usually seen as a poor loser.

There is, in fact, a strong tendency in most of us to focus on successes and ignore defeats, at least in others if not ourselves. We also unwittingly focus our attention on things that agree

The politics of contradiction

Politicians who say contradictory things often perversely maintain people's trust. This seems to be because many voters unwittingly self-select the statements that match their own beliefs. They justify to themselves that the politician 'really' thinks the belief that they most want them to have. This effect can be amplified further if their sources of news are also biased in a similar way.

The brain naturally wants to make sense of things, even if they are inexplicable, which means we grant the benefit of the doubt where none is in fact merited. We also don't like to admit we are wrong, so we double down on our original opinions, even when evidence starts to amount that we may have been misled.

with our beliefs, and ignore those that go against them. It's important to be aware of this tendency, so we can remind ourselves to stop and think critically about what we're reading, or hearing.

Dealing with mistakes

From time to time, we all make mistakes, and how we choose to deal with them can in turn convey a great deal to others about our competence. How we perceive those errors can also have a significant effect on our self-confidence.

First of all, it's always worth considering whether it's necessary to point out an error, if it has not yet been noticed. If it would be perfectly reasonable not to have spotted the mistake, and it doesn't cause any problems you can't easily fix, perhaps you shouldn't point it out. If there's nothing to gain, keep it to yourself.

Other times our mistakes are immediately apparent to others, and so a quick, one-time apology is appropriate. If you're late to a meeting, for example, or you make a mistake that directly affects someone, it's good to say sorry. Usually the apology will be accepted, and you can move on.

But apologising can also have its downsides. Firstly, it can put the idea in other people's heads that you are unreliable or incompetent. And secondly, it can help remind them – and therefore reinforce the memory – of your mistakes.

In particular, saying sorry draws attention to the thing you are apologising for. If the person you are apologising to is already focused on your mistake, apologising makes sense. Conversely, if you apologise to someone who is *not* thinking about whatever you are apologising for, you will be drawing it to their attention again. So apologise just once, and don't spend too long on it – a simple 'sorry' is almost certainly fine. And then, once you've apologised, don't bring it up again – ever.

Over-apologising

Some people have a tendency to over-apologise. We know that memories are made stronger by repetition, so every time you apologise again for the same mistake, you are simply reinforcing the memory of your error. In the vast majority of cases, the other person will soon forget the mistake – unless you keep reminding them by repeatedly apologising.

So, for example, if you are late to a meeting, apologise briefly when you arrive. You don't even need to give an excuse, unless you are ridiculously late. Then, when you leave the meeting, there is a very natural tendency to apologise once again – but if you do this, all you are doing is *reminding* them that you were late. They then leave the meeting remembering how annoyed they were that you were late, which they had otherwise completely forgotten.

Don't worry about being judged

We are all a bit self-obsessed – but that's not a surprise. We spend all our lives inside our heads, so of course we focus on ourselves more than other people focus on us. As a result, we tend to overestimate how interested other people are in us, when the truth is that they are *also* busy thinking more about themselves than they are about us.

Have you ever worried that everyone will stare at you if you arrive late at an event? Or have you ever wondered whether other people will think you're strange if you get up on a train and move to a different seat? If so, you're perfectly normal, but the truth is rather disappointing: most of us are so wrapped up in ourselves, we rarely pay detailed attention to other people. We might pay peripheral attention – look up, perhaps – but we soon return to our own thoughts.

The vast majority of the time we are far less obvious, and of far less interest to others, than we assume. Even if someone *is* judging you, there's nothing you can do about it. We can control only our own lives, not those of other people, and ultimately, we must make the decisions that *we* think are right, rather than being unduly influenced by others.

Healthy decisions

Ultimately, enjoying life is about focusing on what's important – and avoiding worry about what's not. Over a long life it can be easy to collect regrets and disappointments, or even sometimes bad feelings towards others. These may all be justified, but ultimately, if they aren't benefitting you, and especially if they are leading to unhappiness, it's best just to let them go. Remember that long-term unhappiness will lead to lasting changes in your brain, impairing learning and leading to other problems.

Sometimes we find ourselves waiting for other people to change, or to apologise for something. But, if they are doing exactly the same in reverse, there will never be a resolution. Ultimately, while we can wish all we like for other people to do things in the way we would want, the only thing we can really control is ourselves – so it's up to us to be the change we want.

And, if it makes it easier, remember that letting go is not the same as forgetting.

Confidence puzzles

All of the following puzzles might appear to require unusual skills, but in truth they can all be solved by a bit of persistence borne of self-confidence. Believing that you can do them – or at least begin to understand them – is all that is required.

No Four in a Row

This puzzle is all about persistence. The rules are simple, since you merely need to fill each empty square with either an 'O'

or an 'X'. You must do so in such a way that no lines of four or
more 'X's or 'O's are formed anywhere in the grid – not even
diagonally. It might sound simple, but the difficulty of spotting
the next move can sometimes cause you to doubt your ability
to complete it. It can also be surprisingly hard to spot potential
diagonal lines of shapes.

One technique that is worth exploring, should you become
stuck, might seem counterintuitive: guessing. In other words,
consider trying a move and seeing if it pans out. If it does not,
you've learned from the guess and can confidently write the
alternative option into the box where the guess originated. This
approach works particularly well on this puzzle, since there are
only two possible options for each grid square.

1

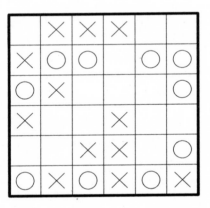

Now that you're familiar with the rules, try this larger puzzle.
You won't need to guess – there's always somewhere that an 'O'
or an 'X' is required in order to avoid forming a line of four or
more of the same symbol.

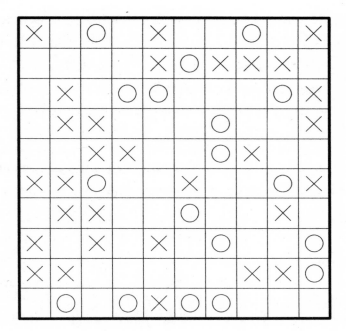

Childlike learning

As children, we learned by repeatedly experimenting and seeing what happened – or in other words by a process which as an adult we might call 'guessing'. Conversely, as we grow older, most people start to become afraid of making mistakes, or of being judged by others for not knowing what to do – so we stop experimenting.

Faced with a grid of many empty squares, it's tempting to decide you don't know what to do and to simply to give up, rather than actually guess and see what happens. The worst-case scenario is that the puzzle doesn't get solved, but then that's clearly no worse than not even *trying* to solve it.

Ultimately, even if someone *were* to judge you for making an incorrect guess, part of dealing with ageing is gaining the ability to discard unimportant opinions and focus on what we know is most important. As we've seen, it's better to make a guess and get the mental experience of seeing what happens, rather than simply not gaining that experience at all.

Fences

In fences, the aim is to draw a loop that visits every dot exactly once each – and that's it! You can join dots using only horizontal or vertical lines, and the loop can't cross over or touch itself.

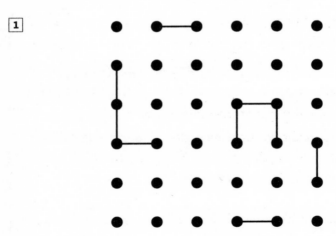

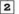

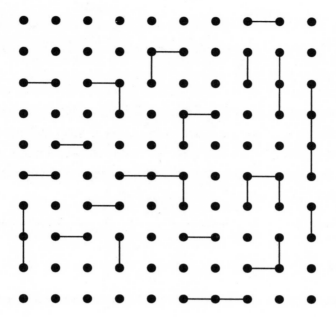

Slitherlink

This oddly named puzzle also involves drawing a loop, and has reassuringly simple rules that nonetheless lead to surprising complexity: just join some (but not necessarily all) of the dots to form a single loop, made up of horizontal and vertical lines, that passes by each number the given number of times. For example, the loop should pass by a '3' on exactly three of its four sides, or by a '1' on just one side; it shouldn't pass by a '0' at all.

Slitherlink is definitely a puzzle that rewards experimentation. It can seem initially baffling, so you will probably find that the easiest way to learn to solve it is via guessing – but then, were you to try several of these puzzles, you would soon start to spot the patterns that can help you crack them more quickly.

1

```
  3   0    3
3   2    2 2
2 3 1 2    1
3   1 3 2 3
1 2   3    1
0   3   0
```

2

```
2 3 1   2 3 1    1
2 3   1     3 2    3
2   2    2 2      2 1
1 3   2 2 2    3 0
2   0   2 2      3 3
3 1     2 2   0   2
  2 3   3 2 1    2 1
3 2     2 2    3    1
1   2 1     2    1 3
  0   2 3 1   2 3 2
```

Numberlink

Here's another puzzle that rewards experimentation. In numberlink, the aim is to draw a set of paths to connect each pair of identical numbers, with one path per number pair. This means that there should be a path from '1' to '1', another from '2' to '2' and so on. The paths cannot touch or cross, and only one path can enter any square. Paths can't travel diagonally.

[1]

				1		
		2			**3**	
		4	**5**			
		1			**4**	
3					**2**	
5						

2

		1						
	2	3						
			4					
	5				6			
	1							
			2					
	7							
				8				
				5		8	4	
	9	7		9	6		3	

Fitword

Finally, on the next page, is a simple word puzzle that you might have tried as a child, but with a grid where there is no immediately obvious 'first move'. The only way to solve a puzzle like this is via initial experimentation. The rules are simple: place each word into the grid once only, crossword style (so they read either across or down in a run of white squares).

STAY SHARP!

3 Letters
Aim
Auk
Cat
Huh
Lad
Mat
Nee
Pal
Run
Tee
Tie
Tot
Yam

4 Letters
Amid
Amok
Apse
Camp
Easy
Emir
Gyro
Hilt
Magi
Mayo
Only
Roti
Sire
Zinc

5 Letters
Aleph
Itchy
Onion
Ready
Reiki
Snake

6 Letters
Guilty
Insist
Patina
Phylum
Random
Remark

Summary

In this chapter we've looked at the importance of staying positive, and why you should take whatever steps you can to deal with sources of long-term unhappiness. We looked at some methods of cheering yourself up, and saw how the good news is that most people tend naturally to feel more positive as they age.

We considered the placebo effect in some detail, and saw how powerfully it demonstrates the importance and effectiveness of positive thinking. We also looked at how it can be exploited by some alternative medicine therapies.

Next, we looked at confidence, and in particular self-confidence, and considered how easily it can be swayed. We considered ways to appear – and actually be – more confident, particularly in front of other people. Feeling more confident can be a key part of feeling more positive.

We saw how people naturally tend to both notice and remember the things that best match their own preconceptions, and how easy it is for our brains to jump to conclusions based on incomplete information. We also considered how we should deal with mistakes, and talked about how important it is to be sensible when apologising, and not to overapologise.

We concluded the non-puzzle part of the chapter with some notes on how we tend to be more occupied with our own thoughts than those of others, and looked at how making healthy decisions in life means relying on our own thoughts and actions. Finally, we introduced several puzzles that all required a certain degree of confidence to solve.

In brief

- Staying positive is important.

- Unhappiness and stress is damaging, and changes our behaviour.

- Physical exercise, laughter, listening to music, and social contact can all help cheer you up.

- We tend to become generally happier as we age.

- The placebo effect means we can sometimes feel better simply because we *expect* to feel better.

- Alternative medicine has its limitations and should not be relied upon for treating serious illnesses.

- We have every reason to be confident in ourselves and it's good to come across as confident to others.

- People tend to remember successes in others, not failures.

► We shouldn't go out of our way to point out our own flaws.

► It's not a good idea to over-apologise – it makes it too memorable.

► Other people are generally less interested in you than you think(!).

► Confident persistence can sometimes help solve puzzles.

► Guessing/experimentation is a powerful solving technique.

Coming up

In the next chapter, we'll take a closer look at concentration and focus – and how you might go about improving them – as well as covering some tips for helping to avoid distractions.

7 Concentration and Focus

Have you ever noticed how the hardest part of a task is often getting started? You really want to tidy the attic, or write to your sister, but somehow you never get around to doing so. Or perhaps you often start to do something but get distracted and struggle to complete it.

Everyone has the same problems from time to time, with starting on a task and then maintaining focus, so in this chapter we're going to look at what you can do when you're struggling to concentrate on a task. We'll cover getting started, and then look at maintaining focus, before moving on to various puzzles that all require focus and concentration to solve.

Your brain

There's a lot going on in your brain all the time, some of which occasionally intrudes into your conscious mind, and we have a number of different senses that we can't just 'switch off' – so it's no wonder that it's easy to get distracted.

We aren't capable of consciously thinking about more than one thing simultaneously, so every time you are distracted – and are trying to pay attention to more than one thing – you are switching your attention back and forth between tasks. We've already seen how limited your short-term memory is, so you tend to lose the thread of your thoughts when this happens. At best, it simply makes you less efficient.

Properly concentrating on a task can be difficult at the best of times, therefore, but after the age of 40 it starts to get harder and harder. Our brains become less good at switching between tasks, so even slight distractions make it more likely that we will lose our concentration. It becomes more important to take extra steps to help ourselves maintain our attention, if we wish to be able to complete tasks efficiently.

All the attention in the world isn't going to help if you've not actually started on a task, however, so let's start by looking at some tips for getting going.

Getting started

With any task, you have to pick what it is you're going to do first. In some cases this won't require much thought, or may be entirely prescribed, but for more open-ended tasks it can sometimes feel overwhelmingly complex. Writer's block is an example of one such obstacle, where the need to 'get going' requires so many decision to be made that it becomes difficult to know where to start.

Luckily, there are various techniques that you could try to help you get started on a problem or activity:

► Break complex tasks down into lots of smaller tasks. If those are still too intimidating, break them down in turn. If you are trying to come up with a plot for a novel, for example, make a list of decisions that you could make separately: work out where it is going to be set; when; with what characters; for which audience; and so on. You might change all of these decisions later, but making smaller, less momentous decisions can help to get you over that first 'getting started' hurdle.

► Think about where you would like to end up, once you have completed a task. What steps would you need to work *backwards* from that state to where you are now? This isn't relevant to every task, but it can sometimes help break a problem down. Thinking about it from a different angle can lead to realisations you might not otherwise have had.

▶ Jump into the middle of the task, if that's practical, rather than starting at what you think of as 'the beginning'. Try something out, even if you don't know what the result will be. Just like solving a puzzle by experimentation, you can often make progress on a task by making some initial guesses and seeing what the effect is. These methods work well for artistic endeavours, or in situations where decisions can be undone if they don't work out.

▶ Maybe you are being too ambitious? It's great to aim high, but being realistic is also sensible. Is the task too broad, or the decisions too open? Start with a simpler aim, and you can always pivot to a more complex aim later, once you have a better idea of how to reach it – or have completed the initial task. It's better to start with a short story than a novel, for example. Ambition is fantastic, but it's also really satisfying (and good for your brain!) to complete a task. This method also has the benefit of letting you make your mistakes on a more limited task first, leading to better results as you move on afterwards.

▶ If there is a creative decision holding you back, try simplifying it arbitrarily. Instead of painting *any* picture, for example, decide that you are only going to consider painting a picture of the first thing you see that you like when you flick open a magazine.

▶ It's fine to aim for perfection, but don't waste time trying to reach it. It's better to finish something, rather than to set such high sights that you can never complete a task. In almost all aspects of life, good enough is all that is required. For example, when you get directions from one place to another, all you require is for those directions to be sensible and accurate. They don't need to be a perfect route, even if you could define 'perfect' in any case.

▶ Discuss how to get started with other people. Even someone who has no specialist knowledge can often make sensible observations, or can trigger a thought that has not previously occurred to you. When you get too close to something, you can't always see the big picture.

▶ Discuss the task with *yourself*. This might sound strange, but explaining – out loud, to yourself – what you plan to do, or need to do, can really help. When we speak out loud we use different parts of our brain, and the need to form a coherent explanation requires us to think about tasks from a different angle. This often enables us to spot flaws, or potential solutions, that we hadn't previously seen.

Once you have come up with a strategy for getting started, and are ready to focus, the next step is to remove any potential distractions that could keep you from making progress.

Distractions

What are the likely distractions that might break your focus on a task?

Make a list of the things that often distract you, and see if there's anything sensible you can do to minimise them. This might mean muting a phone, disabling email fetching, or something as simple as closing a door or window that is letting in a draught or noise. It could also mean asking people not to disturb you unless it's urgent, and removing anything from your field of view which you know is prone to take your attention.

If you are easily distracted by sounds, consider replacing noisy devices. While our brains will often eventually tune out repetitive sounds, such as background chatter, more occasional sounds – such as noise from a keyboard that clicks loudly as you type, or a chair that creaks as you write – could take you out of the moment and distract you from the task in hand, especially if you are already finding it difficult to concentrate.

Another possible distraction is hunger. If you find yourself easily distracted around meal times, work after you have eaten, or try to minimise any distracting food smells. It can also be hard to concentrate in a room that's too cold, hot or draughty, so do what you can to resolve these issues first.

Finally, try to clear your mind of other thoughts that might distract you. There are probably other things you need to do too, so make a list of all of the non-task-related things that are on your mind. Getting these down on paper will mean you don't need to worry about forgetting them, and it will allow you not to be distracted by the sudden remembrance of them along with the thought that you must be sure not to forget them. It's a surprisingly powerful technique for such a simple step.

Distractions with age

When we are distracted by something, it can be very hard to switch our attention back. This effect becomes even more significant as we age, to the point where some elderly people will literally just forget about the task they were previously engaged in, when distracted. This effect is similar to how we once were as toddlers, when we could be made to completely forget some upset simply by being presented with a new activity to try.

Focus

After taking reasonable steps to eliminate likely distractions, and having worked out how to start, you then need to maintain your focus while you are working on a task. When we lose focus, we often also lose track of our thought process, and may need to revisit several steps before we can continue – and we might struggle to get going again too, significantly slowing us down.

Start by writing down a plan for a session, and give yourself a list of smaller targets to aim for. What these are will depend on the task, but if you were writing, it could be a certain number of words, or it could simply be to have spent an hour concentrating on the task. You can use these targets as points where you will take a break or reward yourself in some way (even just with a cup of tea), since it's often a lot easier to keep going on a task when you know a break is coming up. Also, be sure to set yourself targets that you are realistically able to meet so you don't set yourself up for frustration.

Realistic targets help motivate us to keep going, reducing the chance of distractions. If you decide that you won't be finished until some part task is complete, you can focus on just that section of the project with the knowledge that you will be 'done' soon. It also means that you feel a sense of satisfaction when you reach your target, rewarding you for the progress you have made. This in turn makes it easier to focus next time, since your brain will look forward to the pleasurable feeling of reaching your targets.

Attention

Try to notice when your attention is wavering. If you realise you are having trouble concentrating, deliberately take a break. It's better to have a chance to relax, so you can continue when you feel more ready to do so, than to struggle and make little or no progress. You are also giving your unconscious mind a chance to carry on thinking about the problem. If you reach an impasse, try sleeping on a problem – this can sometimes really help, as we'll discover in the next chapter.

If you know that you have trouble paying attention for a sustained period, build in appropriate breaks in advance, rather than aiming for longer sessions which are hard to complete. You could also experiment with different lengths of break, too – perhaps 10 minutes is all you need, but maybe you need an hour or more before you are ready to continue. What works best for you might change over the years, too, so don't be afraid to change the way you tackle tasks to adapt to your changing brain.

Concentration and focus puzzles

These puzzles all require a certain degree of persistence to complete, but will reward those who are willing to focus and pay attention. Try the following puzzles and see how you get on.

Dominoes

Draw lines along the dashed borders to form a complete set of 28 dominoes, with one of each value of domino. Use the check-off chart to keep track of which dominoes you've placed. One domino is already marked and checked off for you, to show how it works. A '0' represents a blank on a traditional domino.

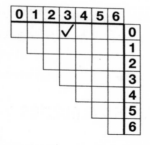

Number path

Write a number in each empty square so that the grid contains every number from 1 to 25 once each. You must place the numbers so that you create a path that visits every number from 1 to 25 in increasing numerical order. The path can travel only horizontally or vertically between touching squares, without leaping over any squares.

5				1
	7		13	
		9		
	21		11	
25				17

King's journey

If you've solved the number path puzzle above, try this much-trickier variant. The rules are the same but now you also have the ability for the path to travel diagonally between squares, as well as horizontally and vertically.

CONCENTRATION AND FOCUS

1 Place 1 to 25:

		8		
	2		7	5
		1		25
16				24
17	15		20	21

2 Place 1 to 36:

	4	1		26	28
6			32	33	34
		17		36	
		8	18		
	12			19	21

3 Place 1 to 64:

3						48	
1			58	53	50		
	6						
	8			26			44
	9		28		62	40	42
	19						37
		13	30		64		
			32				

Code-breaker

This puzzle can be solved simply via persistence, so it may test your ability to focus.

Every letter in each of the following sentences has been shifted through the alphabet by the same amount, relative to its correct position in the alphabet. For example, if each letter has been shifted forward by a single place, A has been changed to B, B has been changed to C, and so on right through until Z has been changed to A.

See if you can work out what shift has been applied to this famous Shakespeare quotation, so that you can reveal the original phrase:

1   Gd ksqga zc rfc dmmb md jmtc, njyw ml.

Here's another encoded Shakespeare quotation, which uses a different shift:

2   Ukxobmr bl max lhne hy pbm.

And here's another Shakespeare quotation, with a different shift again:

3   Ftqdq ue zaftuzs quftqd saap ad nmp, ngf
            ftuzwuzs ymwqe uf ea.

Mini number grid

This puzzle looks like it might be simple to complete, but it can take some persistence to solve. The fundamental rule is to place each number from 1 to 9 once each into the grid. But:

- ► If there is a white circle between two neighbouring squares, they must contain consecutive values, such as 3 and 4, or 7 and 8.

- ► If there is a black circle between two squares, the value in one must be twice the value in the other, such as, for example, 2 and 4, or 3 and 6.

▶ If there is *no* circle at all, neither of the above is true – the numbers are not consecutive, and neither is twice the value of the other.

See how quickly you can complete each of these grids. They might take longer to solve, and therefore require greater focus, than you would predict.

[1]

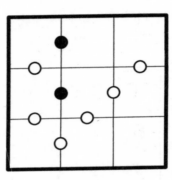

[2]

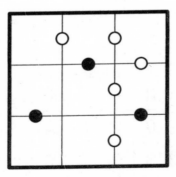

rrows

his puzzle is all about making slow, methodical progress. The
ıles are simple, but the puzzle is not. To solve it, place one
rrow in each dashed-line box, so that every arrow points either
p, down, left or right, or at one of the four main diagonals.
he arrows must be placed so that each solid box has the given
umber of arrows pointing directly at it.

3	6	1
8	4	3
2	4	0

2	4	7	5
0	2	3	4
3	0	2	3
2	2	1	1

Maze

As a final concentration challenge, try this elaborate maze. There's nothing particularly tricky apart from its size, but you'll need to pay attention in order not to lose your place while travelling through these tiny corridors!

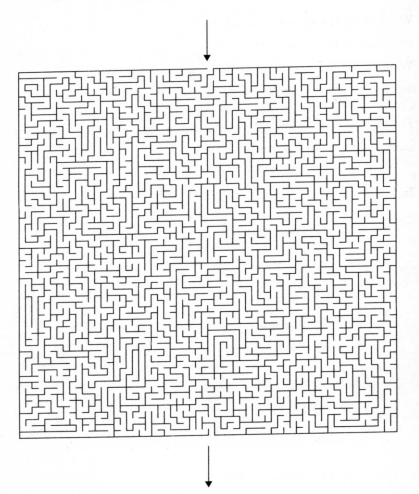

Summary

In this chapter we've looked at the difficulty in maintaining focus on a task, and on gaining that concentration in the first place. We saw how easy it is for our brains to get distracted, and how this tendency gets worse as we age.

We looked at various methods to help to get started on a task, and then considered various ways of minimising distractions. We also considered ways to help maintain focus, including setting targets and scheduling breaks.

Finally, we concluded with a selection of puzzles that all required sustained concentration to solve.

In brief

- ▶ Concentration gets harder in later life.

- ▶ Get started on a task by splitting it into simpler challenges.

- ▶ Experimentation is a good way of getting past a sticking point.

- ▶ 'Good enough' is usually all that is required, not some notion of perfection.

- ▶ Consider discussing problems with others – and yourself.

- ▶ Try to minimise distractions to help maintain focus.

► Make notes of any other tasks that might distract you before beginning a task where you need to focus.

► Set realistic targets, including small goals if appropriate.

► Once you get started, try not to switch attention until you reach your target time or goal.

► Build in breaks, if necessary, when working on a project.

Coming up

In the next chapter, we'll take a closer look at the various day-to-day things you can do to help look after your brain, ranging from physical exercise and a healthy diet through to meditation.

8 Looking After Your Brain

We all know we should look after our bodies, and if we fail to do so, the effects are often quite noticeable. We struggle to walk up slopes, or become tired after relatively short trips. Our appearance may change.

What's much more hidden, however, is the effect that a lack of physical fitness has on our brains. Scientists now know that, as we age, maintaining a keen level of physical fitness is a significant component in maintaining good mental health. In other words, being fit and healthy can help counteract many of the mental effects of ageing, and decrease your risk of developing dementia. So you owe it to yourself to do what you can to look after your health – not just for the rest of your body, but for your brain too.

Physical health

As we saw earlier in this book, from our mid 20s onwards, brain cells start to die, in a process that gets faster and faster the older we get. The *only* way we currently know to counteract any part of this is by ensuring we get regular sustained aerobic exercise. This exercise helps your brain to generate new neurons in the hippocampus (see page 27), allowing it to replace significant quantities of those that are lost as a natural effect of ageing.

It's therefore of critical importance to your mental well-being to take regular exercise no matter your age, particularly in terms of your memory. Put another way, sitting still all day is a bad idea, and will accelerate the decline of your brain.

Exercise

The best exercises to help your brain are aerobic activities, such as walking, running, cycling, rowing, swimming and skipping. The longer you can sustain the exercise for, the better.

Research has suggested that other common types of exercise, such as weight training or interval training, do not have the same neuron-creating effect, although they may have other benefits. It's still the case that any exercise is better than no exercise, so better to do something you enjoy than nothing at all.

The precise effectiveness of aerobic exercise does vary from person to person, but greater physical fitness also carries other benefits. Being fitter and healthier increases the flow of oxygen to the brain, meaning that you can replenish the supply of energy to your neurons more quickly than a less healthy person would, literally allowing you to think faster.

Further brain benefits of exercise

Physical exercise also makes it easier to concentrate after the exercise, and fitter people generally report less trouble maintaining focus.

Even a small amount of movement can help with focus, so if you ever find your attention wavering, you could stand up and wave your arms around, or pace up and down a room for a few minutes, to help you regain your focus on a task. There is also evidence that exercise helps you to be creative, perhaps by allowing you to relax and your unconscious mind to come up with its own ideas.

Exercise also helps relieve anxiety, reduces stress levels, and has even been shown to have a small effect in helping to deal with depression. It generally makes you feel better about yourself, too, which is always good for your brain.

Interestingly, it's also been shown that you can learn more efficiently during moderate exercise. So next time you want to remember something, visit a gym and pop on a treadmill while you read all about it! (Best not to try reading while walking or running along a pavement.)

Last, but by no means least, exercise also helps protect against other diseases that can be damaging for the brain, such as the high blood sugar levels which can result from diabetes.

A sensible diet

Exercise should go hand in hand with a sensible diet, so that your brain is getting the nutrients it needs.

In chapter 2 we discussed the chemicals which the brain requires, and talked about what food might be good for your brain. More broadly, however, there is no specific set of miracle foods when it comes to diet. What works well for one person, in terms of maintaining a healthy body, may not work for another – we are all different because of our genetics and our personal histories.

Eating habits

Some advice is relevant for almost everyone:

- ► Eat breakfast. Most studies agree that you will eat less healthily if you miss breakfast, and doing so is very unlikely to help you lose weight if that is your aim.

- ► Avoid temptation by not keeping supplies of biscuits, cakes and other unhealthy foods to hand. These may be fine in moderation as part of a balanced diet, but it's easy when you're tired (or feeling low) to eat them to excess.

▶ If you tend to eat too much, try using a smaller plate so less food looks more visually filling. Also, wait five or even 10 minutes before getting an extra portion – it takes your brain time to realise that you are no longer hungry.

▶ If you get hungry between meals, have a few nuts, an apple or some other sensible snack. This will often reset your brain's desire for food without involving overeating. Try portioning them out in advance – while you are full – if you find yourself over-snacking!

▶ Drink more water. Sometimes when you feel hungry you are actually thirsty, and water is a healthier alternative to many other drinks. That said, don't worry about having specific amounts of water each day – you will naturally drink the water you require, without having consciously to monitor your water intake.

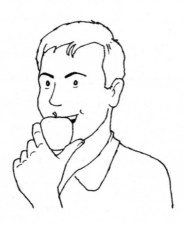

Diet tips

In terms of *which* foods to eat, here are a few key tips:

- ▶ The most basic rule: eat a varied diet. Don't have the same small set of meals over and over.

- ▶ Aim to have more fruit and vegetables – but minimise juices, which release their sugar far more quickly than their corresponding whole fruit.

- ▶ Choose less processed, higher-fibre foods where possible, such as wholemeal bread, brown rice and wholewheat pasta – and make sure you have plenty of fibre in your diet in general.

- ▶ Minimise heavily processed, pre-prepared foods, which often contain undesirable preservatives as well as fewer nutrients than their original ingredients. This can also apply to many takeaway or restaurant meals.

- ▶ Include fish as part of your diet if you can, once or twice a week – particularly oily fish.

- ▶ Avoid foods that are high in fat, salt or sugar, and choose unsaturated over saturated fats.

- ▶ Make sure you have sufficient protein in your diet, such as meat, fish, eggs, beans, pulses and so on. If you eat meat, limit your intake of red and processed meats.

It's generally also wise to avoid fad diets that might be recommended from time to time by various authors – these are often based on at best circumstantial evidence rather than solid scientific research.

Stress

We all feel stressed from time to time. It's a perfectly natural part of being human, and absolutely nothing to worry about so long as it goes away again. But what if stress hangs around, and you rarely get a break from its effects?

Brief periods of stress can be stimulating, but if it continues for too long, it starts to be debilitating. Long-term stress changes your brain's behaviour, placing you in a permanent fight-or-flight situation where you don't act in the same way you otherwise would. This means that learning is impaired, since your brain's focus is elsewhere. It also makes paying attention to a task considerably harder.

Stress also has a range of physical effects, including making you more prone to illness. If you find yourself regularly feeling stressed, you should try to do something about it, including potentially seeking professional medical advice. There are various treatments and therapies that may help you.

Chronic stress (long-term stress that feels out of your control) can even permanently damage your brain, so it's really important to tackle sustained sources of stress as soon as possible – or try to find a way to cope with them if they are truly unavoidable. This may of course be very hard to achieve, but it doesn't change the facts – if you don't deal with it, chronic stress will permanently damage your brain.

If someone you know is suffering from chronic stress, they may have given up hope of ever being able to avoid it, and might take some persuasion to seek out professional help – but seek out help they should.

Drugs

A drug is a medicine or other substance which has a physical effect on you when you eat, drink or otherwise absorb it. Even those intended to be beneficial can have unwanted effects, so all drugs should be treated with respect.

Recreational drugs

Recreational drugs – including alcohol and nicotine (found in tobacco) – generally cause effects which are not well understood, but one thing we do know is that they all work by affecting your brain chemistry and, in turn, your behaviour. This means that recreational drugs may have potential mental dangers beyond any damage they can also inflict on other parts of your body. Alcohol, for example, has been shown to damage the connections between brain cells if taken in excess – as well as its more well-known role in damaging your liver. When *not* taken in excess, however, various studies have suggested that small amounts of alcohol can actually be beneficial for your health.

Too much caffeine?

Even caffeine, as found in coffee, tea and some other drinks, may have negative effects, since too much may lead to confusion, headaches, a rapid heartbeat, increased blood pressure, an increased need to urinate and various other ailments. In the elderly, too much caffeine contributes to bone brittleness, so in old age you may need to reduce your caffeine intake. What's more, suddenly reducing your caffeine intake can also lead to an unpleasant range of withdrawal symptoms.

Medicines

Medicinal drugs can carry their own risks, but normally the benefits will far outweigh these risks. Even so, it's rarely wise to start on a new drug just before you go to bed, in the unlikely case you have a bad reaction.

Sometimes the side effects of certain medicines are not well understood, and can vary from person to person. If you start experiencing unexpected changes in your mood, behaviour or sensations after starting on a new medicine, it is worth considering whether the medicine might be the cause – but always talk to a doctor before stopping any course of medication, since the effects of stopping may be far more problematic than any side effect.

Depression

It's not uncommon for people to feel depressed when they are suffering, either from an ailment or from a loss. But what if you start to feel depressed seemingly without reason, or stay that way for long periods of time? It can be extremely debilitating, not to mention hugely unpleasant.

Clinical depression – serious, persistent depression – hugely impacts on quality of life, and can lead to a wide range of physical and mental problems, including a rapid deterioration in your general health. As a result, professional medical treatment should always be sought as soon as possible.

Depression in later life

Unfortunately, depression can often fail to be diagnosed in later life since the symptoms can sometimes be dismissed as simply the inevitable effects of ageing – even by ourselves. It's important to be aware of this fallacy, since depression in older people should be actively treated, just as it would be for a younger person.

Indeed, some people will start to struggle with depression only in later life, when changes in their situation contribute to a feeling of hopelessness. As a result, we may not always realise what is happening to us.

The risk of depression also becomes a considerable problem once people enter care homes, with some studies reporting that as many as two in five residents are affected. With over 400,000 people in care in the UK, that's a staggering number of people, but it's not hard to see why those in this situation might start to feel hopeless about the future. But, just as in any situation, this type of depression must be treated.

Symptoms of depression include:

- ▶ a lack of interest in what's going on around you;

- ▶ the loss of enjoyment in activities you once preferred;

- ▶ unexpected tiredness;

- ▶ loss of appetite;

- ▶ impatience and irritability;

- ▶ feeling that you are a burden to others;

- ▶ spending a long time dwelling on long-gone problems, or relatively small issues;

- ▶ wishing you were no longer alive.

Depressed people typically won't have all of these symptoms, and may indeed have only one, so if you think that you or someone you know may be suffering from depression, you should always insist on a professional diagnosis and then treatment – it is a show of strength to ask for help, not weakness.

Keeping things fresh

If you eat a healthy diet and do what you can to maintain your fitness, there's no reason why getting older should be a cause of any great concern. Indeed, one of the most important things you can do is carry on planning for the future.

We saw earlier in the book how important it is to challenge yourself continually. If you have settled into a routine where you do many of the same things each day, make a conscious effort to break out of it and challenge yourself with something new.

It's never too late to try new activities and in Western countries with ageing populations there's never been a greater variety of organised events to choose from – and these bring the benefit of extra social contact. No matter what age we are, we nearly always benefit from contact with other people. Trying new activities might take effort, and involve stepping outside your comfort zone, but the effort will repay you many times over. Perhaps you'll enjoy them, or perhaps you won't – but you can always stop and choose something else, and you'll never know until you try.

Don't fear change

Whatever our age, it's always worth considering making major changes in our lives, even if they seem daunting. So, if you think there are changes you can make to improve your life, act now! Don't wait for some future day that may never come – and remember, every time you put something off it gets easier to put it off again the next time. Maybe you've often wished to move nearer to other members of your family, or to a house that better suits your current needs. If so, don't wait for a 'perfect' time to do it – it may never arrive.

Be sure to plan for the future, just as you did when you were younger. Having things to look forward to, or upcoming events to give you a sense of purpose – and of the passing of time – is important. Even if you are suffering from ill health, try and keep your life as varied as possible.

Sleep

Everybody sleeps, and yet we know so little about it. What we *do* know is that it is absolutely essential. If you don't sleep, you will die – but long before that you will be severely impaired. You will find it incredibly hard to focus, and will have trouble controlling your thoughts.

In particular, your brain needs you to sleep. Sleep is when it performs its daily housekeeping, going through the experiences of the day and consolidating what it has learned – so sleep is therefore important for forming lasting memories. This probably accounts for some aspects of our dreams, as we run through our experiences in ways that don't correspond with our usual experience of reality.

Your brain also has plenty of time to think while you sleep. This is why you can sometimes wake up and find the answer to a problem, or a new idea, suddenly presenting itself – either immediately, or later in the day. We know that your brain uses just as much energy while you sleep as it does when you are awake, which gives some indication of just how much is going on while you sleep.

Sleep needs

Your sleep needs will change as you grow older, but no matter how old you are, it's always important to make sure that you get proper, regular sleep. If you find yourself unable to sleep, speak to a doctor. There can be many causes, and you may be able to receive treatment. If you were to continue to not sleep properly, a wide range of health problems could ensue. That said, the odd sleepless night is of no special concern, beyond the temporary annoyance and tiredness it brings.

Find out how much sleep you should be getting for your age, and aim to make sure you achieve it. Until later life this tends to be a minimum of seven hours per night, although it can vary by an hour or so from individual to individual. Very few people can get by on substantially less.

Mindfulness and meditation

If you have trouble relaxing, you might try meditation, or mindfulness techniques based on meditation. These are simple exercises you can perform to help you to calm a busy mind. Some people use them at the start of every day, while others do so at the end of each day to prepare them for sleep – or, of course, at other times too.

These techniques work by helping to calm conflicting thoughts, leading to a more relaxed physical state. This in turn is more conducive to being able to focus, or to get to sleep more easily. They don't work for everyone, but if you find that your mind feels 'busy' and full of distractions, you could try a basic exercise for five or 10 minutes and see if it helps.

Some meditation techniques involve various intricate methods to enter trancelike states, but simply sitting still, somewhere quiet, and focusing on breathing calmly and gently can be effective. Close your eyes, rest your hands on your legs and pay attention to only your breathing for a few minutes. You could play some gentle music in the background, to add to the calming effect, if you wish. Try and empty your mind of thoughts, and sit quietly and peacefully in the moment.

Calmly praying, if appropriate for your personal beliefs, can also have a similar effect, as can simply sitting peacefully in a church or other place of worship. Blocking out the rest of the world, and focusing on universal truths, can help your body relax and feel better able to deal with the problems of the outside world. There's nothing wrong with 'letting things go' for a bit, and it may help make you more effective for the remainder of the day.

As an alternative to meditation, simply finding time for yourself might be all you need. Perhaps you have some private space you can go to where you won't be disturbed. If so, spending a few moments relaxing there quietly might just give you a moment to catch your breath, and recharge your mental batteries.

Hearing loss

Hearing loss can affect people at any age, but it's natural for hearing to get worse with age. This can be annoying in its own right, but because some decline is natural then we might not always realise if our own hearing has become much worse than it should be for our age.

Poor hearing is certainly an annoyance, but untreated hearing loss has been linked to an increased risk of dementia, so it's important not to ignore it. If you have any doubts about your hearing – for example, if you turn the TV up much louder than you used to, or regularly miss details in conversations because you can't hear clearly – be sure to have your hearing checked by a doctor. Your brain will thank you for it.

Relaxing, creative puzzles

We've covered a range of topics in this chapter, so it's time to relax with some gentle puzzles.

Although many of them involve being creative, they are designed so that no matter how artistic you think you are – or aren't – you can still have a go.

Square grid

Colour in some of the squares in this grid to reveal a hidden picture of your own choice. It could be an abstract pattern, or it could be a simple blocky drawing. Some examples are included to give you inspiration, but there's absolutely no requirement to create anything like them.

There are no right answers, so even if you just shade alternating columns to create a simple pattern, that's okay! Most people find it pretty relaxing to colour in squares, so as long as you don't feel any pressure to create some kind of masterpiece you should find this calming and relaxing. And who is to say what a masterpiece is or isn't, anyway?

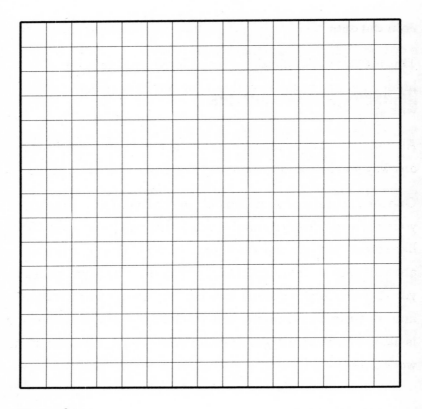

Examples

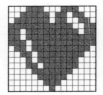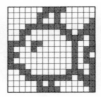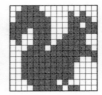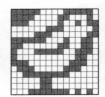

Join the dots

This is a dot-to-dot puzzle with a difference: there is no hidden picture, beyond anything you might come up with yourself!

All you have to do is join some pairs of dots. You can do this in any way you like, and without any need to use all of the dots.

One idea is to start by joining dots at random. Then, after you've joined a few, you might realise that it's starting to look like something – maybe a face, or a wonky building, or just an abstract pattern. If so, great! Carry on joining, until you decide you're done. Or, if it doesn't look like anything, join a few more and check again. No matter how you join the dots, the end result is likely to look visually interesting. And hey presto – an instant work of art!

Poetry posers

Have you ever written a poem, or wanted to? Well, poet or not, this activity is for you.

The aim is simple: supply the second line of a couplet, to make a short (two-line!) poem. It could rhyme, if you wish, perhaps in an amusing way – but it doesn't have to. Again, there is no right or wrong answer.

1. ▶ Every single day I wake and find,

    _____

2. ▶ I wandered through the park today,

    _____

3. ▶ Leaves float by in patterned whirls,

    _____

4. ▶ The immemorial seasons flow,

    _____

What's in the box?

This is a more open-ended drawing task. The aim is once again simple – to decide what's hiding inside each box.

The outside of each box is shown, but what's on the inside? That's entirely up to you! Draw in whatever you think is there.

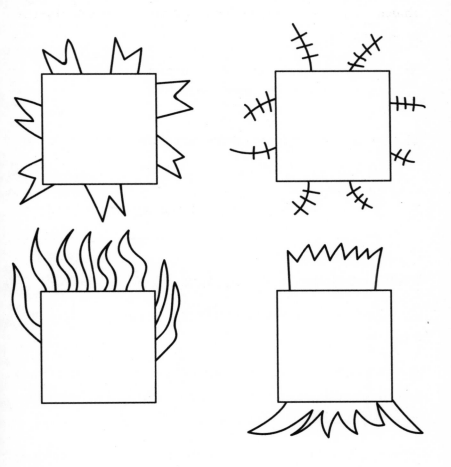

Acronym action

Here's another poetry-based task. In this one, however, you are given only the first *letter* of each line. Can you supply the rest of each line to create two short verses?

1 A _____

   C _____

   E _____

   G _____

2 B _____

   D _____

   F _____

   H _____

Missing punchlines

This creative task involves providing the missing punchline for some jokes.

There are once again no correct answers, so it's all about coming up with your own ideas. But – if you've ever pulled a Christmas cracker – you'll know that almost anything can pass for a joke …

If you are stuck, feel free to replace the questions with some joke prompts of your own.

1 ▸ Why did the donkey cross the road?

_____

2 ▸ What happened when the short dog ran into the
long grass?

_____

3 ▸ Did you hear the one about the misprinted newspaper?

_____

4 ▸ What do you call a one-legged dinosaur?

_____

Puzzles to sleep on

These puzzles involve abstract thought, so they are all ones that
might be solved by sleeping on them. So, if you can't think of
a suitable answer, maybe your unconscious mind will come up
with one while you sleep! Return to the puzzle the next day and
see if inspiration strikes.

Riddles

Each of these riddles involves some simple trick or play on
words in order to provide a suggested solution that is given in
the Solutions chapter. You might, of course, come up with your
own answers that are just as good as those given at the back.

1. Where does eight always precede seven, and seven precede three, and yet two still follows one?

2. What word begins with E, ends with E, and yet can have any number of letters within it?

3. Which word is always spelled incorrectly in the dictionary?

4. What is it that the more you take, the more you leave behind?

5. What occurs in every second, twice in a decade, but not once in a century?

6. There is something that everyone has, but which is used by others far more often than themselves. What is it?

7. I am bought for eating, and put on the table for a meal – but am never eaten. What am I?

8. What is it that can go straight through glass without breaking it?

Lateral thinking

In these puzzles, the aim is to come up with an explanation for the situation, or to answer a question with a possibly unintuitive answer. In some cases there may be more than one perfectly good answer.

1. A man walks past 20 unrelated families and they all say 'Hello, father!' How is this possible?

2. A woman is sitting indoors with the lights off, and without a fire, match, torch or similar, and yet she is able to read a book with no difficulty. How is this possible? Can you come up with *three* completely different explanations for how this might be?

3. A man falls off a 40-foot ladder that is leaning against a building, and is uninjured except for a small bruise. Given that he landed on solid concrete, how is this possible?

4. A woman is sitting indoors reading a book. When she looks out of her window she can't see anyone, but passers-by can see her. How is this possible? It is normal, two-way glass in the window.

5. A scientist knocks a glass beaker off a tall counter and the beaker falls to the floor – but not a drop of liquid is spilled. Why not?

6. An on-duty police officer sees a bus driver travelling the wrong way up a one-way street but does nothing. Can you think of a reason why?

7. A woman is trying to move a box of her possessions into her new office, but the box won't fit through the door. There are no other windows or ways into the room. How

does she solve her problem, without dismantling any part of the office?

8. A woman can't sleep, so she calls her neighbour in the middle of the night. She hangs up after a few rings, before he answers, and then falls asleep. Why does she do this, and how does it help?

Summary

In this chapter we've looked at how important it is to look after our brain properly. We considered the importance of physical health, and how it is critical to maintaining mental health as we age. We looked at the types of exercise you should aim for, and then moved on to consider diet and eating habits.

Next, we considered stress, and saw how debilitating chronic stress can be. We also looked at drugs, and considered some common sense approaches to both medicine and recreational drugs such as alcohol.

We talked about depression, and how it may go undiagnosed in later life – and how common it is in those in care homes. We also looked at ways to keep your routine fresh, and why getting older is not an excuse to stop planning for the future and pushing forward with bold changes.

Moving on, we took a look at the importance of sleep, and why you can't live without it. We also considered meditation and mindfulness, and saw how they can be useful for some people to help them relax. Finally, we took a look at why progressive hearing loss can cause more problems than you might imagine.

We then concluded the chapter with some relaxing, creative puzzles, followed by some puzzles that you might well find easier to solve once you've slept on them!

In brief

- ► Physical exercise is essential to look after your brain.

- ► Sustained aerobic exercise is best of all.

- ► Exercise also helps you concentrate, and reduces stress levels.

- ► Exercise can even help you learn.

- ► Eat breakfast, and strive to have a sensible diet throughout each day.

- ► Chronic stress can damage your brain, impair learning and make you prone to illness.

- ► Medicines and drugs may have side effects on your brain, so look out for unexplained changes.

- ► Depression may be less likely to be diagnosed in the elderly, and in particular can be triggered by a move to a care home.

► Consider making major changes you would like in your life now, rather than waiting.

► Always continue to make plans for the future.

► Do what you can to ensure that you have regular, sufficient sleep.

► Your brain needs sleep, and can carry on thinking while you sleep.

► Try quiet meditation to help calm your mind.

► Don't ignore hearing issues – have them checked out by a doctor.

► Creative tasks can be a great way of relaxing.

Coming up

In the next chapter, we'll take a look at life skills in general, including managing expectations, and remembering to look out for yourself. We'll also consider some useful ideas to help keep your brain active as you move on from the activities in this book.

9 Life Skills

Life is a journey, but we don't always know where it's heading.

We might aim for a destination, but take a detour along the way. So long as we don't get lost, does it really matter where we end up? No matter where you are now, there's still time to set out on a new path.

In this chapter we'll take a look at why deciding what you want to do is not as simple as we'd sometimes hope, due to the multi-layered structure of your brain that we learned about in chapter 1. We'll also consider the route you've taken through life, and why some aspects of your journey might have been more heavily influenced by others than you realised. We'll look at expectations, and consider in detail some of those new paths that you could start exploring right away.

Competing impulses

Have you ever known that you were full, but still really wanted to keep eating anyway? If so then that's to be expected, and it's all down to the structure of your brain – and the way it links to your body – that we looked at back in chapter 2. In the case of diet, a more primitive part of your brain tells you to keep eating, since it hasn't yet received the stop signal, while a more evolved part tells you that really you can't still be hungry and that it's a good idea to stop eating now.

Given that your brain has competing circuits, with different parts arriving at different decisions, this means that it really does argue with itself over what to do. Controlling your more basic impulses will often involve a genuine test of willpower, of gut desire versus a more level-headed analysis.

Slow thinking

The parts of your body that are controlled via chemicals in the bloodstream are much slower to respond than those connected to the central nervous system, which are controlled via the electrical impulses that flow through it. Knowing how your brain works, and how it communicates with your body, allows a better understanding of how to take control of your life – so it's you pulling the strings, and not some reflexive animal instinct.

Distant thoughts

Did you know that physical distance from your brain can affect your speed of reaction? This is why a short amount of time can pass between realising that you have stubbed your toe and then actually feeling the associated pain. It takes time for the signal to make its way from your toe all the way up to your brain!

Separate regions

The complex nature of your brain, with many aspects of your cognition divided among different areas, also means that different areas might reach different conclusions at the same time. Parts of your vision circuitry might decide that you're looking at a hole in the ground, for example, but another part of your mind might find elements that cause you to wonder whether you are actually just looking at a spill of black paint. So which part of your brain makes the final decision? Well, that might just depend on how much conscious attention you're paying.

Unconscious thoughts and decisions

The way that your brain has evolved means that you still have many parts of it in common with less advanced animals. Just as they are able to react to their environment without a higher-level consciousness of themselves, so the less evolved parts of your brain also react instinctively. This means that you can sometimes find yourself doing things that you didn't consciously decide to do.

These lower-level responses also mean that you sometimes do things that are absolutely *not* in your best interests. Freezing with fear in the face of danger is an unhelpful response if you spot a car speeding towards you; no matter how great an idea it might have been when facing down an angry animal, it will rarely serve you well in the modern world. And, as morbid as it may sound, this is one reason why it might be wise to prepare for potential life and death situations by thinking through what your response would be. Having a plan should such a situation ever arise might help your conscious mind to override your more primitive responses, potentially saving your life. It's also why you should pay attention to safety announcements.

Herd instincts

Your unconscious responses are often based on herd instincts. For example, people start to doubt themselves – even if they initially felt sure of something – if they hear a number of other people say or do something contradictory to their initial belief. Once *enough* people start saying that same thing, we may even start to believe it, no matter how ridiculous it may once have sounded.

Another herd instinct is that we tend to physically follow groups of people, even if we think they are going the wrong way or doing the wrong thing. We also suppress our own sometimes strong desires in order to avoid the fear of acting in a way *others* might think is odd. Even if our desire is to leave a building when a fire alarm continues to ring, when the conflicting desire to stay in order to fit in makes little or even no sense, many people will still remain inside rather than risk going against the 'herd decision'. Unfortunately, if everyone is copying everyone else, the fire alarm will be completely ignored – at least until something else happens that prompts them to re-evaluate their decision.

Failing to evacuate

In life-and-death traumatic events, some people's brains become so overwhelmed that they go into neurological shock. This prevents them from thinking clearly and it can be fatal. In one aircraft collision, the roof was ripped off a plane as it sat on the runway. Many of the passengers stayed sitting as if glued to their seats and failed to evacuate. Those whose brains were able to cope with the immediate trauma, and make their way out of the plane, survived.

Embrace your inner child

Controlling competing impulses is just one of life's many challenges. A much more general one is exploring the greater arc of our lives.

As we journey through life, we may not end up exactly where we once expected, but along the way we pick up a valuable toolkit of skills and experiences which – if we care for our brains – will continue to expand throughout our lives. Indeed, one of the most important lessons of this book is that you should continue to challenge yourself throughout life and not be afraid to act with a childlike wonder for the world around you.

When you were a child, you had no trouble asking for what you wanted, and didn't worry about what other people would think of you when you tried something and it didn't work out. If you got on a bike and promptly fell flat on your face, you still tried again almost right away. But then, when you became an adult, the chances are that this optimistic approach to life became suppressed. This is because we suppress those desires that we think others would consider childish – and we are often time-poor too. But now, in later life – at last! – we might once again have the chance to experience some of the same freedom we had as a child. We perhaps have time, and less concern about what others will think. And if not now, then when?

As we age, we are more likely to have both the time and the means either to try something new or to engage with a hobby that we were never able to commit to before. If you have always wanted a large doll's house, or an expansive train set, then maybe now is your chance. Don't limit yourself by what you think are the expectations of others. You only have one life, so live it.

Expectations of others

Some people spend their lives suppressing their own desires in order to fit in with others. Putting aside the inevitable sacrifices and compromises in living with other people, and raising families, it isn't healthy to *completely* suppress your own needs. But even people who think they make their own decisions tend to have been heavily influenced by the people around them – even when they don't realise this has happened.

Academic subjects

Perhaps we were once told that we weren't very good at maths, or someone criticised our writing, and it left a mark on our younger psyche that has never quite gone away. The truth, of course, is that we all have at the very least some basic talents in these areas, and yet our entire lives can then be influenced by the casual uninformed comments of others many years ago.

It's never too late to break free of the limitations that others have imposed on you, whether they did so unwittingly or not. If maths has always challenged you, practise doing simple mental arithmetic (such as adding up a restaurant or shopping receipt), or play an online maths game; or if you feel your writing has always been a weakness, why not take a course in creative writing? The chances are that you have considerably more abilities in these areas than you might once have been led to believe, and have laboured under a misapprehension for much of your life.

Creative subjects

It's not just academic skills, either, that can limit us. Some people consider that they 'aren't creative', or 'aren't artistic', but that's simply not true. Any able-bodied person can pick up a brush and flick some paint on a piece of paper, and hey – that's art! It's easy to confuse the ability to draw a photorealistic scene, which is indeed an impressive talent, with the fundamental creative, artistic abilities that we all have. Indeed, as we've seen, your brain is inherently acting creatively all the time.

Art is not just about being able to draw something precisely. It is about creating something new, whether that comes from your imagination or the random vagaries of a brush flick. So why not take up painting, or sculpting, or any other creative activity? The creative puzzle activities at the end of the previous chapter hopefully helped to demonstrate just how easy it can be.

Music

For many people, music is one of the great escapist experiences of life. It has the ability to transport you somewhere new, or to change your mood in just a few minutes. It's also a fantastic experience for the brain if you make your own music, so, if you play an instrument, make sure you keep it up if you can, and why not take up a second instrument too?

If you don't play an instrument, try learning one – it's never too late. The piano is a great choice, and with modern electronic keyboards you don't need as much space as a traditional piano – plus you can play without disturbing anyone else. The guitar is another popular choice, and is neither expensive nor particularly large. Or you could even take up drumming – perhaps with an electronic kit that can be listened to with headphones! Whatever you choose, don't miss out on trying because someone once led you to believe that you weren't very musical, or because you simply never tried it. Find a local class or teacher to get you started.

If you are already an experienced musician, try a new style of playing. If you usually play classical, try pop or jazz. If you can't play by ear, try to learn. If you have always wanted to compose music, now's your chance. Modern computer systems can do such a good job of emulating any instrument that you can hear your composition right away, should you fancy channelling your inner Beethoven.

New puzzle challenges

This book has a wide range of puzzles to help provide diverse new challenges, but they are just the tip of the iceberg. There are many books of mixed puzzles available, often with titles that include the words 'brain training' or 'brain games'. Look for them in the puzzle-book section of shops (sometimes called 'Indoor Games'), and not in the self-help or popular psychology sections.

There are also many different types of physical puzzle that you might enjoy, from jigsaws onwards. Perhaps the most famous of these is the Rubik's Cube, which is capable of providing a challenge to even the smartest minds. Why not give it a go, if you never have, or try it again if you last picked one up in the 1980s!

If you live in a major city, you are likely to have 'escape rooms' in the vicinity. These are venues which provide a series of puzzles that must all be solved in the space of an hour (or thereabouts), and which you are encouraged to tackle as part of a team that you usually assemble yourself. They involve a fun but intensive period of creative problem-solving, as well as generally a small amount of light physical exercise, so they are a great experience to try if you are able. Generally, the hosts will provide hints to help you out while you play, so they can be enjoyed no matter the extent of your puzzle-solving skills.

Tougher challenges

Many experiences in life require a combination of skills, so look for a varied range of activities to take part in. Remember that those things providing the greatest mental challenge are also the ones that will be best for your brain, so don't just stick with the tried and tested but look out for the unexpected and new too. If you're an artist, try learning how to write computer code; if you're an accountant, try creative writing. Pick something outside your existing experience to ensure a challenge.

All this said, it's important to know yourself, and know what you can physically do. There's no point hurting yourself with impractical tasks, or trying something that could put you at real risk. But, conversely, have self-belief, and don't skip things just because they seem hard. Your brain has an incredible range of skills, and you owe it to yourself to use them.

All-round puzzles

The challenges below are a great place to start, since they all require a range of skills to solve. They will test a variety of your abilities – and require a mix of different types of thinking – to complete.

If you get well and truly stuck on one of these puzzles, don't be afraid to steal a quick look at the solutions to get you going. You can even copy part of the solution back onto the puzzle to get you on the right track. There's nothing wrong with doing this, and it's better to make progress than get to the point where you simply give up.

Skeleton crossword

This crossword is a much tougher challenge than a regular crossword, since most of the black squares and clue numbers are missing. It's up to you to restore them as you solve the crossword.

The finished puzzle is rotationally symmetrical, so if the square two across from the left on the top row is shaded, then the square two across from the right on the bottom row will be too. Solution lengths and a few initial placements are given, which will also help you get going.

If you start this and find it too tricky, it could be a good puzzle to collaborate on with someone else. On this kind of task, two minds can often be better than one – especially to help avoid making incorrect assumptions. With this sort of puzzle, it's easy to become convinced something must be true when in fact it was actually just a guess.

LIFE SKILLS

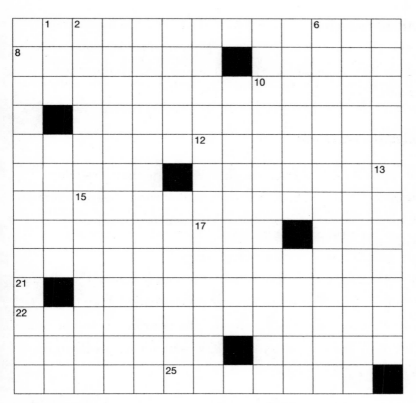

Across

1 Large, colourful bird (7)
5 Store (4)
9 Seat containing storage space (7)
10 Accepted practice (5)
11 Theatrical play (5)
12 Most infrequently seen (6)
14 Covered area with shops (6)
16 Sustained fight between armed forces (6)
18 Scattered untidily (6)
19 Fuming (6)
22 Commence (5)
23 Try (7)
24 Stench (4)
25 Teach (7)

Down

2 Minor actor (5)
3 Biblical law (11)
4 Middle (6)
6 Public transport (7)
7 Watery part of milk (4)
8 Fruit-flavoured drink syrup (7)
10 Not practical (11)
13 Keepsake (7)
15 Small, country house (7)
17 Without a salary (6)
20 Confess (5)
21 Former Russian ruler (4)

Outside sudoku

If you're used to solving your sudoku puzzles with the starting numbers inside the grid (and who isn't?), this puzzle adds a twist to that by beginning with the starting numbers *outside* the grid.

Each of the numbers given outside the grid belongs somewhere in the nearest three squares in its row or column, but it's up to you to work out which one. If there is more than one number shown for a set of three squares, remember that they are not necessarily placed in the grid in the given order.

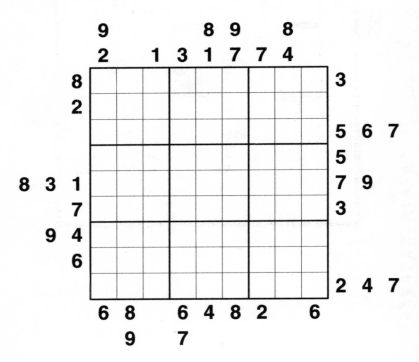

Pipeline

Draw a section of pipeline in every empty square to form a single loop of pipe that visits every square at least once.

In each square, the pipe can either pass straight through, make a 90-degree turn, or cross directly over itself. Some segments are already given.

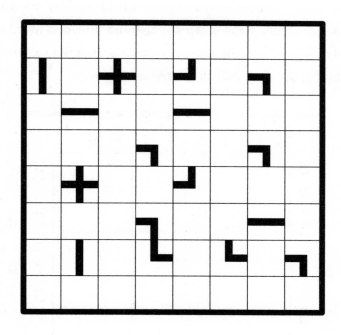

Loop sweeper

In this puzzle, the aim is to draw a single loop that passes through the centres of some (but not necessarily all) empty squares, travelling only horizontally or vertically between squares. The loop can't revisit a square, so it can't cross over or touch itself. It can't enter a square with a number.

Numbers in some squares show precisely how many touching, including diagonally touching, squares that the loop must visit. For example, the '4' at top left indicates that *exactly* 4 of the touching squares are visited by the loop.

4				7		6	
				8			
							3
5		6		7			
							2
				4			

Killer sudoku

This puzzle is much easier if you are already familiar with sudoku, so if you've never solved sudoku before then this will be a particularly tough challenge!

The aim is to place a number from 1 to 9 into each blank square, so that every number appears once in each row, column and bold-lined 3x3 box. The grid must be filled in such a way that all of the numbers inside each dashed-line region add up to the total given at the top left of that region. Furthermore, you can't repeat a number within a dashed-line region, so a total of '6' could be made by 1, 2 and 3, but never by 1, 1 and 4.

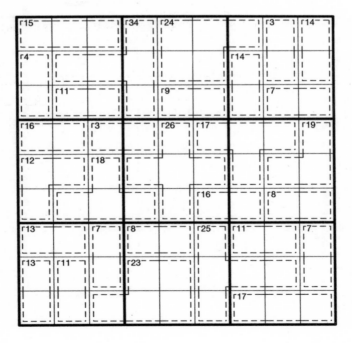

Spiral crossword

The crossword opposite is not as tricky as some of the puzzles in this section, but due to its unusual format it can seem quite confusing nonetheless! The clues here are not given in the usual across or down way, but run either inwards or outwards around the spiral. Each word should be placed in the set of numbered boxes shown next to the clue, running in the appropriate direction. Every numbered box therefore forms part of two words – an inwards one, and an outwards one.

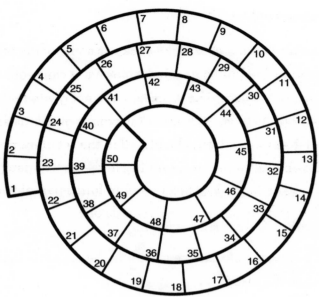

Inwards

1–6	Married
7–9	Ball's target?
10–14	Noble gas used in some lamps
15–23	Apprehending
24–26	Sharp bite
27–29	Unprocessed
30–33	Wooded valley
34–38	Church keyboard
39–45	Alarm
46–50	Divisible only by itself and one

Outwards

50–47	Arab ruler
46–43	Attack with thrown objects
42–40	Type of rodent
39–36	Glitch
35–30	Wheeled
29–23	Distorting
22–19	Possible hair infestation
18–16	Get it wrong
15–12	In a short while, poetically
11–4	Lengthened
3–1	Dawn grass deposit

Written logic puzzle

In this puzzle, the aim is to make a deduction by reading all of the clues. An accompanying grid provides an easy way to keep track of eliminations – place an 'x' when you know that two options do not go together, or a tick if you are sure that they do.

There are three women: Beatrice, Lucy and Maria. One of them is aged 29, one is 32 and one is 43. One is a doctor, one is a lawyer and one is a teacher. You also know the following three facts:

► Maria is older than the lawyer.

► The 29-year-old's name is later in the alphabet than the teacher's name.

► Beatrice's age is an odd number.

What is the name, age and occupation of each woman?

| | Age | | | Occupation | | |
	29	32	43	Doctor	Lawyer	Teacher
Name Beatrice						
Lucy						
Maria						
Occupation Doctor			
Lawyer			
Teacher			

Name	Age	Occupation

Sudoku 3D Star

In this final puzzle, the aim is to place a number from 1 to 8 in every empty box so that each row, column and bold-lined 2×4 or 4×2 region contains eight different numbers. The rows and columns follow the bends of the 3D surface, so there are a total of 24 rows plus columns in this puzzle.

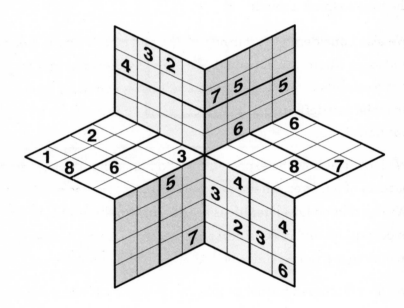

Summary

In this chapter, we've taken a look at how the structure of your brain can cause you to make decisions that may not always be in your best interests, whether it's having an extra dessert when you're already full, or reacting in an unhelpful, instinctive way to a situation where you would behave differently if you had the time to think about it.

We also considered the journey of life, and how it may not have ended up where you expected. We looked at how important it is to embrace your inner child, and liberate yourself from artificial restrictions that may have prevented you from trying out new things.

We looked at how the expectations of others can influence many aspects of our lives, whether consciously or subconsciously. We considered how later life is a great time to throw out these expectations, and make a new start in a wide range of areas – including art, music and even literature and mathematics.

We also discussed further puzzle challenges, both along the lines of those in this book as well as more physical ones too.

Finally, we concluded with a range of puzzles that required an all-round skill set to solve.

In brief

- ► Competing impulses are a natural part of how our brains have evolved, so sometimes we need to consciously overrule what a part of our brain is telling us to do!

- ► Decisions that our subconscious brains make, based on primitive herd instincts, may not always be to our advantage, so it's important to stay alert and think about what we're doing.

- ► We gain skills throughout life, and should make sure we take advantage of them.

- ► We shouldn't be afraid to try things we've always wanted to do, if we are now able.

- ► Other people's expectations can limit us, so it's important to be true to yourself.

- ► New puzzle challenges, including escape rooms, can expand on the puzzles in this book.

- ► Look for tougher challenges that aren't typical of your usual activities.

- ► Stand up for yourself and take steps to achieve the things you desire.

► Don't give up on tricky tasks, but don't be afraid to seek help if it's available.

Coming up

In the next section, we'll complete your brain journey by briefly reviewing many of the topics that we've covered so far.

Conclusions

Your brain is phenomenally complex. In fact, it's by far and away the most complex machine in the known universe. Little wonder, then, that we are just starting to scratch the surface of how it works – and that so much of it remains a mystery to us.

What we do know about the brain, however, is of real importance. Throughout this book you've learned a great deal about how to look after your brain, and how it is a key component of your body that requires every bit as much attention as your physical fitness.

What we've covered

We started off the journey by looking at your physical brain, and saw how it was structured by being built out of 100 billion neurons with 100 trillion synaptic connections between them, plus more than a trillion glial cells helping to keep everything working. It's hardly surprising that there is so much we don't understand about it, therefore. One thing we can learn from the structure of the brain, however, is why your immediate urges and desires don't always align with the decisions you'd take if you stopped to think about something dispassionately.

We took a look at how your brain changes throughout your lifetime, and how you must keep on challenging yourself in order to help fight against the natural decline in mental abilities throughout our adult lives. We also saw how certain illnesses can affect your brain, and considered what you can do to try and decrease your chances of being affected by them.

Next, we took a detailed look at brain training, and considered how it might benefit you. We discovered that its most significant benefits are in later life, but that the best training of all is to challenge yourself continually, with a wide range of different tasks and activities – including, but not limited to, the types of puzzle found within this book.

We took a deep dive into how your memory works, and why some things are more memorable than others. We saw how we all have pretty much the same fundamental memory capabilities, and it's simply how well we learn to use our memory that distinguishes us from one another.

We discovered just how easy it is for memories to be changed, and how this is likely to happen gradually over time. We also saw just how inaccurate our memory can be, and how we are misled into thinking that our recall of events is far more precise than it typically is.

We looked at a range of techniques to help you learn about a subject, as well as some specific techniques to help with remembering names, lists and facts, and tried out the techniques on a number of exercises.

Challenging your brain is of such importance that we spent some time looking at why this is, and how you might go about doing it, such as by travelling – or by simply experiencing nearby places in a new way. We also looked at how important our language skills are, and how they form a key part of the life-long learning process that we should aim to engage in every day.

We saw how important it is to remain mostly positive about life, and why your brain will suffer if you aren't able to do so. To demonstrate this, we considered what the placebo effect shows us about the power of positive thinking, and considered the influence of confidence – and in particular our self-confidence – on both what we are able to achieve and our own state of mind.

In order to successfully challenge yourself, you need to be able to sufficiently focus on a task without being too distracted, so we considered a range of ways to help you concentrate, and also considered how you might go about tackling a complex task that seems too intimidating to get started on.

We looked at the importance of physical health on our mental health, and saw that it becomes ever more critical, the older we get, to have regular aerobic exercise – along with a healthy diet too, of course. We saw how exercise not only helps our brains directly, but can also help alleviate stress, and we saw why it's so important for your brain that you try to deal with any chronic, long-lasting stress.

We also considered other aspects of your mental health, such as the risks of depression – and why it may be harder to diagnose in older people, despite it being more likely in some cases. We also saw how drugs and medicine can affect our mental state, and how planning for the future is an important part of maintaining a healthy state of mind. On top of that, we also considered how important it is to get enough sleep, and how meditation can be useful in some cases for helping us to relax.

Finally, we took a look at your entire journey through life, and saw how much it might have been influenced by early comments that you took to heart as a child – but remembered that it's never too late to try something new. We also saw that you are likely to have talents you have never appreciated, and why later life gives us the excuse we might have needed to do so.

Next steps

Take advantage of what you now know about your brain to continue to challenge yourself, and fight against age-based mental decline.

Use the tips from the book to help with everyday situations. For example, remember that explaining things to others can help you to look at them from a fresh angle; if you are stuck, sleep on a problem; and make sure you pay attention to, and then practice or repeat again, things you want to remember.

As you carry on through life, stop sometimes and take time to challenge your preconceptions, and don't forget to pause when necessary and think about which default brain responses might not be helpful.

Look out for yourself

Ultimately, the person who knows you best is *you*, so it's up to you to stand up for yourself and make sure that you look after both your body and your brain.

You can't wait for someone else to suggest the things you want to happen – you need to take steps to try and make them happen for yourself.

Concluding thoughts

Our later years should not be consumed with expectations of an inevitable decline, but filled with fresh activities, new social engagements, exciting adventures, expansive learning, and as many new challenges as we can find the time for.

With sufficient exercise, a balanced diet, and some suitable brain maintenance activities, there's no reason – other than the vagaries of ill health – why you shouldn't go on to experience a long, healthy and happy later life.

Solutions

Chapter 4: Memory

Remembering Names and Faces (page 107)

The faces are now in the order of (from left to right, top to bottom) Adrianna, Joe, Edward, David, Patricia and Henrietta.

Connecting Objects (pages 110–12)

There are eight missing objects:

- ► Alarm clock
- ► Bicycle
- ► Bucket
- ► Globe
- ► Leaf

- ▶ Plant pots
- ▶ Pot of pens
- ▶ Wellington boots

Chapter 5: Lifelong Learning

A to Z (pages 137–8)

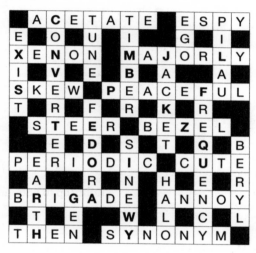

Zigzag (page 139)

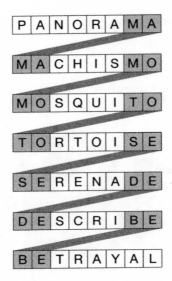

Anagrams (page 140)

Mammals:

1. Elephant

2. Antelope

3. Giraffe

4. Rhinoceros

5. Anteater

Countries:

1. United Kingdom

2. Australia

3. Barbados

4. Mongolia

5. Afghanistan

First and Last (page 141)

1. C: CAUSTIC

2. S: STUDIOS

3. L: LOCAL

4. M: MAIM

5. A: ARIA

6. W: WIDOW

7. E: EULOGISE

8. P: PRIMP

9. T: TAROT

10. R: ROAR

Letter Sequences (page 142)

1. Months of the year in order: January, February, March, April, May, June, July, August, September, October, November, December

2. Colours of the rainbow in order from red: red, orange, yellow, green, blue, indigo, violet

3. Cardinal numbers from one upwards: one, two, three, four, five, six, seven, eight, nine, ten

4. Planets in order outwards from the sun: Mercury, Venus, Earth, Mars, Jupiter, Saturn, Uranus, Neptune

5. Days of the week starting from Thursday: Thursday, Friday, Saturday, Sunday, Monday, Tuesday, Wednesday

6. Fractions in decreasing size: half, third, quarter, fifth, sixth, seventh, eighth, ninth, tenth

7. Scientific classifications in order of increasing specificity: kingdom, phylum, class, order, family, genus, species

8. Elements of the periodic table in increasing atomic number order: hydrogen, helium, lithium, beryllium, boron, carbon, nitrogen, oxygen, fluorine, neon

SOLUTIONS

Initial Letters (pages 143–4)

Novels and their authors:

1. *To Kill A Mockingbird* by Harper Lee

2. *The Great Gatsby* by F. Scott Fitzgerald

3. *Mrs Dalloway* by Virginia Woolf

4. *Brave New World* by Aldous Huxley

5. *The Prime of Miss Jean Brodie* by Muriel Spark

Films:

1. *Gone with the Wind*

2. *The Sound of Music*

3. *Butch Cassidy and the Sundance Kid*

4. *One Flew Over the Cuckoo's Nest*

5. *Close Encounters of the Third Kind*

Shakespeare plays:

1. *Romeo and Juliet*

2. *Julius Caesar*

3. *King Lear*

4. *As You Like It*

5. *Much Ado About Nothing*

Works of art and their creators:

1. *Mona Lisa* by Leonardo da Vinci

2. *The Starry Night* by Vincent van Gogh

3. *Girl with a Pearl Earring* by Johannes Vermeer

4. *Guernica* by Pablo Picasso

5. *The Persistence of Memory* by Salvador Dalí

Word Circle (pages 144–5)

First word circle: the word that uses all the letters is reading (or grained, or the archaic word gradine). Other words to be found include: aged, aid, aide, aired, and, arid, danger, dare, daring, darn, dean, dear, deign, den, die, dig, din, dine, diner, ding, dire, dirge, drag, drain, end, gad, gained, gander, garden, gird, grade, grand, grid, grind, idea, nadir, raged, raid, rained, ranged, read, red, rend, rid, ride, ridge, rind and ringed.

Second word circle: the word that uses all the letters is awestruck. Other words to be found include: askew, awe, awes, caw, caws, craw, craws, crew, crews, raw, rawest, saw, screw, sew, skew, stew, straw, strew, swat, swear, sweat, tweak, tweaks, wake, wakes, war, wars, wart, warts, was, waste, waster, water, waters, weak, wear, wears, west, wet, wets, wrack, wreak, wreaks, wreck, wrecks and wrest.

Word Square (pages 145–6)

First word square: the word that uses all the letters is relocates. Other words to be found include: are, ares, ate, car, care, cares, caret, carol, cat, cater, core, cores, era, ere, eta, locate, locates, lore, orate, orates, ore, ores, rat, rate, rates, relocate, reset, role, roles, sere, set, taco, tar, tare, tares and taro.

Second word square: the word that uses all the letters is praiseworthiness. Other words to be found include: arrow, ewe, ewes, hop, hope, hopes, how, new, owe, owes, pew, piss, port, praise, praises, raise, raises, rope, ropes, row, sepia, sew, sip, thin, thine, tho, trope, tropes, wen, win, wine, wines, worth and worthiness.

Deleted Vowels (pages 146–7)

Flowers:

1. Daffodil

2. Buttercup

3. Geranium

4. Orchid

5. Fuchsia

European capitals:

1. London

2. Paris

3. Moscow

4. Athens

5. Oslo

Every Other Letter (pages 148–9)

Musical instruments:

1. Violin

2. Guitar

3. Ukulele

4. Piano

5. Clarinet

Types of fruit:

1. Orange
2. Pineapple
3. Blackberry
4. Nectarine
5. Peach

Word Prefixes (page 148)

1. Anticlimactic
2. Interaction
3. Postmodern
4. Preamble
5. Superimpose

Word Suffixes (page 149)

1. Abstraction
2. Catchment
3. Numbness
4. Cavernous
5. Wishful

Word Fragments (page 149)

Occupations: Electrician, lifeguard, pharmacist, solicitor and statistician.
Cocktails: Cosmopolitan, daiquiri, manhattan, margarita and mojito.

SOLUTIONS

Hidden Word (page 150)

Colours:

1. Yellow: When in the woods I **yell, ow**ls hoot.

2. Orange: He often looks f**or ange**ls.

3. Pink: Can you s**pin k**nives quickly?

4. Brown: I pluck just one eye**brow n**ow.

5. Red: I want a bette**r ed**ucation!

Numbers:

1. Two: On bank holidays he won**'t wo**rk.

2. One: Easter is an occasi**on E**nglish people may celebrate.

3. Four: We stuf**f our**selves on Christmas Day.

4. Eight: Nothing can outw**eigh t**he joy of summer.

5. Seven: New Year**'s Eve n**icely bids goodbye to December

Codeword (pages 151–2)

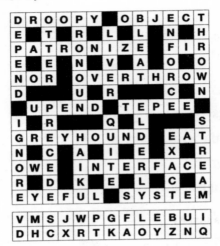

Word Pyramid (pages 153–4)

First word pyramid:

1. ARC
2. CARE
3. CRAVE
4. CARVES
5. SCARVES
6. CREVASSE

Second word pyramid:

1. NUT
2. UNIT
3. UNITE
4. MINUTE
5. MINUETS
6. TERMINUS
7. RUMINATES
8. MINIATURES

Crossword (pages 155–6)

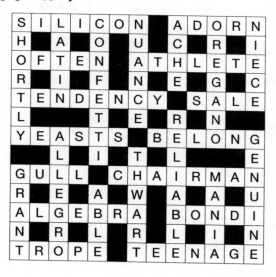

Word Play

1. Shrinking violet

2. Through thick and thin

3. Nothing to it

4. Over the line

5. Fly in the ointment

Chapter 6: Staying Positive

No Four in a Row (pages 175–7)

1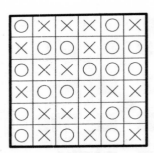

2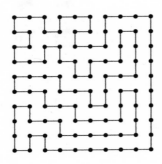

Fences (pages 178–9)

1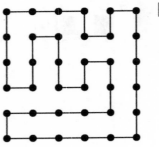

2

Slitherlink (pages 179–80)

1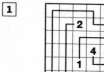

2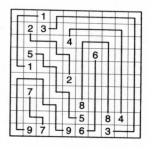

Numberlink (pages 181–2)

1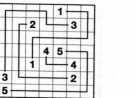

2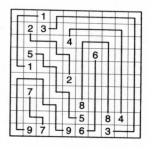

Fitword (pages 183–4)

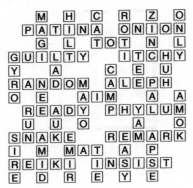

Chapter 7: Concentration and Focus

Dominoes (pages 196–7)

4	3	2	0	4	1	3	3
1	3	0	6	4	6	6	5
2	1	0	3	5	5	1	2
0	6	6	0	3	6	3	4
6	4	3	5	5	1	0	2
2	1	5	2	4	4	2	0
0	6	5	4	1	1	2	5

Number Path (page 198)

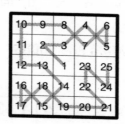

King's Journey (pages 198–9)

1

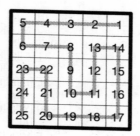

2

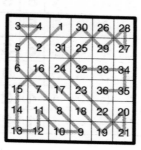

3

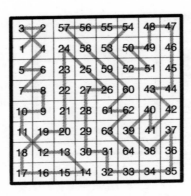

Code-breaker (pages 200–1)

Shift the first quotation forward two letters to reveal:
If music be the food of love, play on.

Shift the second quotation forward seven letters to reveal: **Brevity is the soul of wit.**

Shift the third quotation forward 14 (or backward 12) letters to reveal: **There is nothing either good or bad, but thinking makes it so.**

Mini Number Grid (pages 201–2)

1

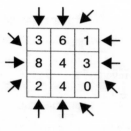

2

7	6	5
1	3	4
2	9	8

Arrows (page 203)

1

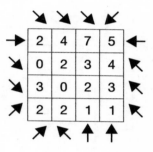

2

2	4	7	5
0	2	3	4
3	0	2	3
2	2	1	1

Maze (page 204)

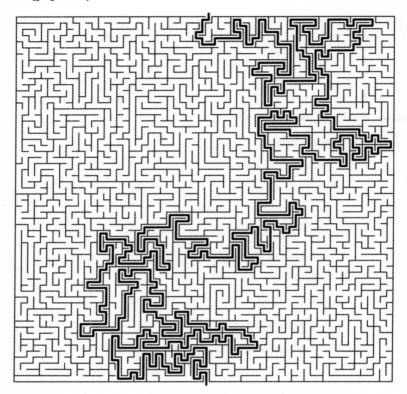

Chapter 8: Looking After Your Brain

Riddles (pages 229–30)

1. In a dictionary

2. Envelope

3. Incorrectly

4. Footsteps

5. The letter 'd'

6. Your name

7. Cutlery and crockery

8. Light

Lateral Thinking (pages 230–2)

1. The man is a priest.

2. It is daytime, so there is light coming through the windows; *or* she is reading on an electronic tablet or other device with illuminated screen; *or* she is blind, and is reading by braille.

3. He falls off a low rung of the ladder, not the top.

4. It is night-time, but the light is on in her room, so she can't see anything outside – but people can see in.

5. The beaker is empty.

6. The bus driver is walking.

7. She takes her possessions out of the box and carries them in one by one.

8. She is being kept awake by her neighbour's snoring, so she rouses him with the phone call until she hears his snoring stop, then is able to fall asleep. This explains the fact that she didn't wait for him to answer.

Chapter 9: Life Skills

Skeleton Crossword (pages 246–7)

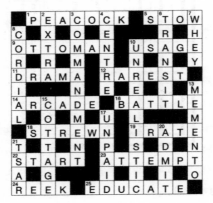

Outside Sudoku (page 248)

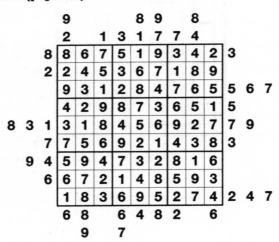

Pipeline (page 249)

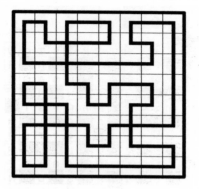

Loop Sweeper (page 250)

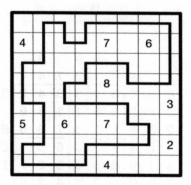

Killer Sudoku (page 251)

2	4	9	6	8	3	7	1	5
3	8	7	4	5	1	6	2	9
1	6	5	9	7	2	8	4	3
9	7	2	1	6	8	5	3	4
4	3	6	5	2	9	1	8	7
5	1	8	3	4	7	9	6	2
8	5	3	7	1	4	2	9	6
6	2	4	8	9	5	3	7	1
7	9	1	2	3	6	4	5	8

Spiral Crossword (pages 252–3)

Inwards			Outwards		
1–6	WEDDED		50–47	EMIR	
7–9	NET		46–43	PELT	
10–14	XENON		42–40	RAT	
15–23	ARRESTING		39–36	SNAG	
24–26	NIP		35–30	ROLLED	
27–29	RAW		29–23	WARPING	
30–33	DELL		22–19	NITS	
34–38	ORGAN		18–16	ERR	
39–45	STARTLE		15–12	ANON	
46–50	PRIME		11–4	EXTENDED	
			3–1	DEW	

Written Logic Puzzle (pages 254–5)

Beatrice is 43 years old and a teacher. Lucy is 29 years old and a lawyer. Maria is 32 years old and a doctor.

Sudoku 3D Star (page 256)

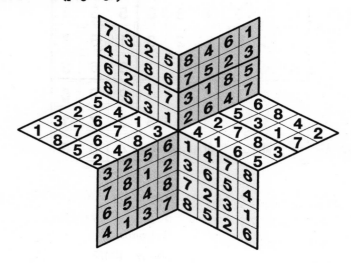

Useful References

The Brain and How it Works

- *Your Brain: The Missing Manual* by Matthew MacDonald (O'Reilly, 2008) – an easy-to-read introduction to your brain, in full colour.

- *The Brain: A Very Short Introduction* by Michael O'Shea (Oxford University Press, 2005) – a pocked-sized introduction in a more academic style.

- *How Your Brain Works: Inside the Most Complicated Object in the Known Universe* by *New Scientist* (John Murray, 2017) – this book introduces the brain from a popular science angle.

- www.nhs.uk/live-well/eat-well – NHS advice on eating a balanced diet.

▶ *Sod It! Eat Well* by Anita Bean and Muir Gray (Bloomsbury, 2016) – a guide to eating well in later life, with solid nutritional advice.

The Changing Brain

▶ *The Brain that Changes Itself: Stories of Personal Triumph from the Frontiers of Brain Science* by Norman Doidge (Penguin, 2008) – a series of stories about the brain's remarkable ability to modify itself.

▶ www.nhs.uk/conditions/dementia – NHS guide to dementia, with information on the signs and diagnosis of dementia.

▶ www.alzheimers.org.uk – the charity Alzheimer's Society, with support and information relating to Alzheimer's disease, including advice for caregivers.

Keeping Your Brain Fit

▶ *Brain Coach: Train, Regain and Maintain Your Mental Agility in 40 Days* by Dr Gareth Moore (Michael O'Mara, 2018) – this book is packed full of exercises to try, along with explanatory text to justify why they are important.

▶ *The Mammoth Book of Brain Games: 365 Days of Puzzles to Keep You Sharp* by Dr Gareth Moore (Robinson,

2014) – this book includes a wide range of types of brain exercise, many of which are puzzles, with a specific exercise or article for every day of the year.

► www.brainedup.com – a daily online brain-training programme I created that can be completed in just 10 minutes a day (a subscription is required for full use, however).

► Peak – a brain training app for iPhone and Android devices.

► The *Sod* series: *Sod Sitting, Get Moving!*; *Sod Sixty*; *Sod Seventy*; *Sod It! Eat Well* edited by Muir Gray (Bloomsbury Publishing). Fitness, mental health, diet and exercise are all covered in these fun, accessible guides to closing the fitness gap and ageing well.

Memory

► *Memory Coach: Train and Sustain a Mega-Memory in 40 Days* by Dr Gareth Moore (Michael O'Mara, 2018) – if you want to practice using your memory, this book is perfect. It contains a hugely varied range of exercises, along with full explanations of many different memory techniques.

► *How to Develop a Brilliant Memory Week by Week: 50 Proven Ways to Enhance Your Memory* by Dominic

O'Brien (Watkins, 2015) – this book covers lots of different memory techniques, giving you more options to pick from for one that works well for you.

Life-long Learning

▶ *Tricks of the Mind* by Derren Brown (Channel 4, 2007) – this extremely readable book covers a range of brain-related tricks, and has useful information on memory techniques.

▶ www.rosettastone.co.uk – a commercial language-learning course provider (paid content required to use).

▶ Duolingo – a language-learning app for iPhone and Android devices.

▶ Memrise – another language-learning app for iPhone and Android devices.

▶ www.oed.com – a word of the day appears on the Oxford English Dictionary site, and a free subscription option is provided to receive it via email each day.

▶ *How to Master the Times Crossword: The Times Cryptic Crossword Demystified* by Tim Moorey (HarperCollins, 2008) – an introductory guide to solving all cryptic crosswords, not just the ones in *The Times*.

► *Chambers Crossword Manual* by Don Manley (4th edition, Chambers, 2014) – an alternative introduction to cryptic crosswords.

Staying Positive

► www.mind.org.uk – Mental health charity Mind provide information and local support for anyone experiencing problems with their mental health.

► www.nhs.uk/conditions/stress-anxiety-depression/ mental-health-helplines – a list of helplines for various mental health issues.

► www.meetup.com – a site for getting involved in new, local social groups.

Concentration and Focus

► *The GCHQ Puzzle Book* by GCHQ (Michael Joseph, 2016) – one of the toughest puzzle books ever published, this is full of extremely hard challenges that often require significant leaps of insight.

► *Enigma: Crack the Code* by Dr Gareth Moore (Michael O'Mara, 2018) – another book that also requires leaps of insight to solve some of the puzzles, but with a much gentler difficulty curve than *The GCHQ Puzzle Book*.

Looking After Your Brain

▶ *Mindfulness: A Practical Guide to Finding Peace in a Frantic World* by Mark Williams and Dr Danny Penman (Piatkus, 2011) – a best-selling introduction to mindfulness techniques.

▶ *Lateral Logic: Puzzle Your Way to Smart Thinking* by Dr Gareth Moore (Michael O'Mara, 2016) – a mix of further lateral thinking, logic and creativity puzzles.

▶ *The Mindfulness Puzzle Book: Relaxing Puzzles to De-stress and Unwind* by Dr Gareth Moore (Robinson, 2016) – a book of gentle puzzles, all designed to be solvable in a short coffee break.

▶ www.ageuk.org.uk – Age UK is a charity providing support and advice for older people. Their website includes tips on maintaining a healthy mind and body in older age.

▶ www.nhs.uk/live-well – health and well-being advice from the NHS.

Life Skills

▶ www.ageuk.org.uk/services/in-your-area/social-activities – Age UK's service for finding clubs and classes in your local area.

▶ www.open.ac.uk – university courses that can be taken via distance learning.

▶ www.musicteachers.co.uk – a website to help you find a local music teacher.

▶ www.puzzlemix.com – my online puzzle site with a range of logic puzzles to solve.

Notes

1 The Brain and How it Works

... one theory suggests Kozliski, James, 'Closed-Loop Brain Model of Neocortical Information-Based Exchange', Frontiers in Neuroanatomy, 10 (3), (2016) – available at https://www.ncbi.nlm.nih.gov/pmc/articles/PMC4716663/ [Accessed March 2019]

... your neurons simply die – and most of them can't ever regrow New cells can be made in many parts of the body by an existing cell splitting into two, but neurons don't have this ability. This means that when a neuron dies, it isn't so easily replaced – and this is why brain diseases can be so debilitating. New neurons can be grown, but only from neural stem cells, and it seems that this will only happen in certain parts of the brain. We also think that long-distance neurons – those connecting distant parts of the brain – can't be regrown.

... injecting vitamins and other supplements Injecting vitamins directly can damage your organs and even your bones, and the procedure itself carries risk of infection, allergic reaction and even air bubbles in the blood (which can be deadly), plus various additional risks if the IV is not correctly placed into the vein. For example, see https://www.nutrition.org.uk/nutritioninthenews/headlines/ivvitamins.html [Accessed April 2019]

... *amounts beyond the RDA* Dangour, Alan D.; Allen, Elizabeth; Elbourne, Diana; Fasey, Nicky; Fletcher, Astrid E.; Hardy, Pollyanna; Holder, Graham E.; Knight, Rosemary; Letley, Louise; Richards, Marcus; and Uauy Ricardo, 'Effect of 2-y n-3 long-chain polyunsaturated fatty acid supplementation on cognitive function in older people: a randomized, double-blind, controlled trial', *The American Journal of Clinical Nutrition*, 91(6) (June 2010) – available at https://doi.org/10.3945/ajcn.2009.29121 [Accessed March 2019]

... *taking extra omega-3 can cause problems* However, you shouldn't have more than four portions a week of oily fish, crab and some specific white fish due to pollutants they absorb from the sea; and shark or marlin should be eaten no more than once a week. For more details, see: https://www.nhs.uk/live-well/eat-well/fish-andshellfish-nutrition/ [Accessed March 2019]

2 The Changing Brain

... *new neurons in the hippocampus* Woollett, Katherine and Maguire, Eleanor A., 'Acquiring "the Knowledge" of London's Layout Drives Structural Brain Changes', *Current Biology* 21 (24–2): 20 December 2011, pp. 2109–2114 – available at https://www.ncbi.nlm.nih.gov/pmc/articles/PMC3268356/ [Accessed March 2019]

... *eating foods with a lower glycaemic index* For an explanation of what the glycaemic index is, see: https://www.nhs.uk/common-health-questions/food-and-diet/what-is-the-glycaemicindex-gi/ [Accessed March 2019]

3 Keeping Your Brain Fit

... *a six-week study of over 11,000 adult participants* Owen, Adrian M.; Hampshire, Adam; Grahn, Jessica A.; Stenton, Robert; Dajani, Said; Burns, Alistair S.; Howard, Robert J.; and Ballard, Clive G., 'Putting brain training to the test', *Nature* 465 (10 June 2010), pp. 775–778 – available at https://www.nature.com/articles/nature09042 [Accessed March 2019]

... *devised by the UK Medical Research Council, the Alzheimer's Society and the BBC* https://www.bbc.co.uk/pressoffice/pressreleases/stories/2010/04_april/20/bang.shtml [Accessed March 2019]

... *a meta study looking for far transfer* Sala, Giovanni and Gobet, Fernand, 'Does Far Transfer Exist? Negative Evidence From Chess, Music, and Working Memory Training', *Current Directions in Psychological Science* (25 October 2017) – available at http://journals.sagepub.com/doi/full/10.1177/0963721417712760 [Accessed March 2019]

... recent study of around 7,000 people https://www.alzheimers.org.uk/research/our-research/have-go-braintraining [Accessed March 2019]

... *that far transfer really does consistently take place* Zelinski, Elizabeth M., 'Far transfer in cognitive training of older adults', *Restorative neurology and neuroscience* 27 (5) (2009), pp. 455–71 – available at https://www.ncbi.nlm.nih.gov/pmc/articles/PMC4169295/ [Accessed March 2019]

4 Memory

... *volunteers became convinced that they had seen Bugs Bunny* Braun, Kathryn A., Ellis, Rhiannon; and Loftus, Elizabeth F., 'Make My Memory: How Advertising Can Change Our Memories of the Past', *Psychology & Marketing* 19 (1) (2002), pp. 1–23 – available at http://scholarship.sha.cornell.edu/articles/332 [Accessed March 2019]

7 Concentration and Focus

... *after the age of 40 it starts to get harder* Fortenbaugh, Francesca C.; DeGutis, Joseph; Germine, Laura; Wilmer, Jeremy; Grosso, Mallory; Russo, Kathryn; and Esterman, Michael, 'Sustained attention across the lifespan in a sample of 10,000: Dissociating ability and strategy', *Psychological Science*, 26(9) (2015), pp. 1497–510 – available at https://www.ncbi.nlm.nih.gov/pmc/articles/PMC4567490/ [Accessed March 2019]

8 Looking After Your Brain

... *helps your brain to generate new neurons* Colcombe, Stanley J.; Erickson, Kirk I.; Raz, Naftali; Webb, Andrew G.; Cohen, Neal J.; McAuley, Edward; and Kramer, Arthur F., 'AerobicFitness Reduces Brain Tissue Loss in Aging Humans', *The Journals of Gerontology*,

Series A, 58 (2) (February 2003), pp. M176–M180 – available at https://doi.org/10.1093/gerona/58.2.M176 [Accessed March 2019]

... *weight training or interval training do not have the same neuron-creating effect* Nokia, Miriam S.; Lensu, Sanna; Ahtiainen, Juha P.; Johansson, Petra P.; Koch, Lauren G.; Britton, Steven L.; and Kainulainen, Heikki, 'Physical exercise increases adult hippocampal neurogenesis in male rats provided it is aerobic and sustained', *Journal of Physiology* 594 (7) (2016), pp. 1855–73 – available at https://www.ncbi.nlm.nih.gov/pmc/articles/PMC4818598/ [Accessed March 2019]

... *a small effect in helping to deal with depression* Cooney, G.M.; Dwan, K.; Greig, C.A.; Lawlor, D.A.; Rimer, J.; Waugh, F.R.; McMurdo, M.; and Mead, G.E., 'Exercise for depression', Cochrane Database Syst Rev. 9 (12 September 2013) – available at https://www. ncbi.nlm.nih.gov/pubmed/24026850 [Accessed March 2019]

... *you can learn more efficiently during moderate exercise* Schmidt-Kassow, Maren; Zink, Nadine; Mock, Julia; Thiel, Christian; Vogt, Lutz; Abel, Cornelius; and Kaiser, Jochen, 'Treadmill walking during vocabulary encoding improves verbal long-term memory', *Behavioral and Brain Functions* 10 (24) (12 July 2014) – available at https://www.ncbi.nlm.nih.gov/pmc/articles/PMC4114134/ [Accessed March 2019]

... *chronic stress ... can even permanently damage your brain* Chetty, Sundari; Friedman, Aaron R.; Taravosh-Lahn, Kereshmeh; Kirby, Elizabeth D.; Mirescu, Christian; Guo, Fuzheng; Krupik, Danna; Nicholas, Andrea; Geraghty, Anna; Krishnamurthy, Amrita; Tsai, Meng-Ko; Covarrubias, David; Wong, Alana; Francis, Darlene; Sapolsky, Robert M.; Palmer, Theo D.; Pleasure, David; and Kaufer, Daniela, 'Stress and glucocorticoids promote oligodendrogenesis in the adult hippocampus', *Molecular Psychiatry* 19 (12) (2104), pp. 1275–1283 – available at https://www.ncbi.nlm.nih.gov/pmc/articles/PMC4128957/[Accessed March 2019]

... *caffeine contributes to bone brittleness* Rapuri, Prema B.; Gallagher, J. Christopher; Kinyamu, H. Karimi; and Ryschon, Kay L., 'Caffeine intake increases the rate of bone loss in elderly women and interacts with vitamin D receptor genotypes', *The American Journal of Clinical Nutrition* 74 (5) (November 2001) – available at https://doi.org/10.1093/ajcn/74.5.694 [Accessed March 2019]

Index

Your Notes

STAY SHARP!

YOUR NOTES

STAY SHARP!

STAY SHARP!

STAY SHARP!

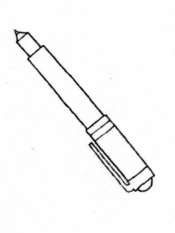